Practising Public Health

A Guide to Examinations and Workplace Application

Practising Public Health

A Guide to Examinations and Workplace Application

EDITED BY

ADAM D M BRIGGS

Wellcome Trust Research Training Fellow
Nuffield Department of Population Health
University of Oxford and
Honorary Specialty Registrar in Public Health
Oxford University Hospitals NHS Trust
Oxford, UK

PAUL A FISHER

Research Fellow in Public Health,
School of Health and Population Sciences
University of Birmingham
Birmingham, UK

ROB F COOPER

Associate Postgraduate Dean and Head of School of
Public Health, Health Education England (West Midlands)
and Honorary Senior Clinical Lecturer
University of Birmingham
Birmingham, UK

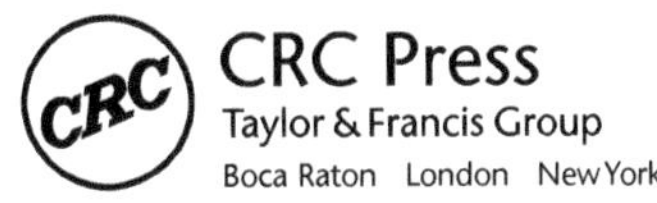

CRC Press
Taylor & Francis Group
Boca Raton London New York

CRC Press is an imprint of the
Taylor & Francis Group, an **informa** business

CRC Press
Taylor & Francis Group
6000 Broken Sound Parkway NW, Suite 300
Boca Raton, FL 33487-2742

Printed on acid-free paper
Version Date: 20151013

International Standard Book Number-13: 978-1-4822-3865-5 (Paperback)

Visit the Taylor & Francis Web site at
http://www.taylorandfrancis.com

and the CRC Press Web site at
http://www.crcpress.com

Contents

Foreword vii
Preface ix
Acknowledgements xi
Contributors xiii
Introduction xv
List of acronyms xvii
List of videos and practising public health tips xix

1 Health protection 1
Paul A Fisher and Nigel Smith
2 Health promotion 21
Val Messenger, Angela Baker and Adam D M Briggs
3 Healthcare public health 45
Christopher Chiswell, Rob F Cooper and Chris Packham
4 Leadership and change management 67
Rachael Leslie and Adam Turner
5 Relevance to public health assessments and examinations 87
Adam D M Briggs
6 Video scenarios 95
Paul A Fisher, Rob F Cooper, Jill Meara and Chris Packham

Glossary 175
References 185
Index 187

Foreword

Public health is about protecting and improving the health of groups of people rather than focusing on individuals as patients.

Public health professionals are involved in preventing ill health, reducing health inequalities and improving the quality and outcomes of health and care services. They must look at the 'bigger picture' and then take action to promote healthy lifestyles, prevent disease, protect and improve general health and improve healthcare services. The population they are working for could be a rural community, an entire city or the global population, but the principles remain the same.

Everyday public health practice involves being able to interact, reassure, negotiate and influence people, organisations and governments. The Faculty of Public Health tests public health practice by a 'show how' exam, the Objective Structured Public Health Examination (OSPHE), Part B of its membership exams.

This book uniquely brings together guidance and video examples of the skills required and practicing public health tips for those taking the OSPHE exam. More importantly, it helps all public health professionals optimise their everyday public health practice in any country dealing with all public health domains (health promotion, health protection or healthcare public health) to better deliver public health and therefore to really make a difference.

It is a most welcome contribution which should enjoy a wide circulation.

Professor John R Ashton CBE
President of the UK Faculty of Public Health

and

Professor Bryan Stoten
Chair of the UK Public Health Register

Preface*

WHY WE WROTE THIS BOOK

This is the book that we would have loved to have had when first practising public health and dealing with people and organisations, and when preparing for the final part of the membership exams of the UK Membership of the Faculty of Public Health (MFPH). When we first started discussing plans for this textbook, we wanted to create something not only to help people sitting Part B of their MFPH exams (the Objective Structured Public Health Examination [OSPHE]), but also to be of practical use to all public health professionals, from both medical and non-medical backgrounds, and including students and more seasoned professionals. With this book, we have tried to provide a guide and a toolbox to help public health professionals make the most of day-to-day interactions in a range of settings with a range of stakeholders – to enable them to maximise their impact on population health. Furthermore, the skills included will help readers to meet the UK Public Health Register practitioner standards and the UK Faculty of Public Health specialty trainee competencies – as such, it complements *Mastering Public Health: A Postgraduate Guide to Examinations and Revalidation*, second edition, CRC Press.

Back in 1995, a professional educationalist's review of the final examination of the Faculty of Public Health in the UK revealed a number of irredeemable flaws, and the faculty's board took the decision that a new faculty examination which was fair and reliable should be developed. Rob F Cooper was asked by the board to lead a team to develop and implement the examination; from start to finish, an objective and reliable exam was achieved within 18 months thanks to the magnificent contributions by many faculty members and fellows. The first sitting of the OSPHE took place in February 1996.

It is an examination like clinical the Objective Structured Clinical Examinations (OSCEs) which role-plays typical occurrences in the practice of public health and requires candidates to demonstrate satisfactory competence in terms of communication skills (presentation and listening), picking up the relevant points of a brief in a timely fashion, making appropriate professional judgements, and dealing with conflict and uncertainty. We are grateful to Chris Packham, who chaired the group which produced the role-play questions, and to Jill Meara, who took over this role when Chris Packham became chair of examiners in 2004, taking over from Rob F Cooper, who had served 5 years. The examples used in this book to illustrate the principles of public health practice are based on real OSPHE questions, which in turn were developed by real public health consultant grade specialists who based the questions mostly on real-life experiences they have had in their public health practice.

BOOK OVERVIEW

The chapters are written to specifically cover the three domains of public health (Griffiths et al., 2005): health protection, health promotion and healthcare public health, including guidance on

* Additional material is available from the CRC website: http://www.crcpress.com/product/isbn/9781482238655.

relevant communication skills. There is also a chapter on leadership and change management and a glossary with examples of how to communicate technical terms in lay language.

Uniquely, we have created a series of videos of genuine MFPH OSPHE scenarios. Along with the scenario packs published in this book, these offer those working in public health, including those preparing for the exam, an insight into what a good – and not so good – performance looks like. The videos provide the ability for the viewer to first score the candidate before comparing their scores to the marks and feedback given by experienced OSPHE examiners. The 'Assessments' section also provides a series of do's and don'ts from previously successful OSPHE candidates.

The book is filled with tips, guidance and exercises covering the practical aspects of working in public health, and we intend it to be used as something that can be dipped into for day-to-day practice, as well as a text that can cover the relevant practical exams and assessments that public health professionals often have to undertake (the introduction provides more on how to use this book). The skills included will be valid in any international public health setting; however, the examples and exercises are developed world focused. This is intentional as it reflects the content of the Faculty of Public Health OSPHE and its related international counterparts. However, despite our best efforts and the support of our external advisory panel, we are aware that the examples are often Anglo-focused and we welcome feedback about parts of the book that may not be applicable to other developed world settings.

THE EDITORS

We count among us not only Rob F Cooper who led the team that designed, developed and implemented the OSPHE, but also Paul A Fisher who was a public health specialty registrar from a non-medical background when he won the McEwen Award for the highest-scoring OSPHE candidate in 2012, and Adam D M Briggs, a public health specialty registrar from a medical background who won the award in 2013. We are hugely grateful to our international advisory panel for helping to maintain the book's relevance to the international public health community, and our individual chapter authors, who have brought their specialist knowledge to the book.

Acknowledgements

The editors are hugely grateful for all the support they have had when putting together this textbook, without which it would not have been possible to complete the project. In particular:

The UK Faculty of Public Health (FPH) of the Royal College of Physicians for providing chapter scenarios, and Bruce Bolam, Linda Garvican, Christine Hine, Adrian Mairs, Jill Meara, Chris Packham, Daniel Seddon and Gerry Waldron, who produced the original scenarios.

Members of the Faculty of Public Health John Linnane and Annette Wood, for helping to mark the scenarios.

Nigel Smith and his media company Cardboard Zebra (http://cardboardzebra.co.uk/) for filming and producing the videos.

The video actors, particularly for their willingness to play the part of poorer performers than they are in order to highlight weaknesses to our audience: Ansaf Anzar, Sally Bradshaw, Carol Chatt, Mamoona Tahir, Dan Todkill, Nigel Smith and Clare Walker.

The UK Public Health Register.

The external advisory panel for providing feedback throughout the project to help ensure that the book is pitched at an appropriate level and for an international audience:

Prof. Charles Guest, Director of Research, Australian Capital Territory Health Directorate, Canberra Schools of Medicine & Population Health, Australian National University, Australia

Dr Ashraf Ahmed Abed Zada, Consultant Family Physician, Chair – MRCGP (Int) Examination Board, Dubai, UAE; Head of Academic Affairs Centre, Dubai Health Authority

Dr YY Ho, Consultant (Community Medicine) (Risk Assessment & Communication), Centre for Food Safety, Food and Environmental Hygiene Department, Hong Kong

Prof. Emer Shelley, Consultant in Public Health Medicine, Health Service Executive, Dublin; Honorary Clinical Associate Professor, Royal College of Surgeons in Ireland

Dr Karen Vincenti, Consultant in Public Health Medicine and Postgraduate Training Coordinator (Public Health Medicine), Office of the Chief Medical Officer, Ministry for Energy and Health, Malta

Dr Stephen Knight, Discipline of Public Health Medicine, College of Health Sciences, University of KwaZulu–Natal, Durban, South Africa

Sir Muir Gray, Consultant in Public Health, Oxford University Hospitals NHS Trust, Oxford, UK

Dr Jill Meara, Deputy Director/Consultant in Public Health, Public Health England, UK

Dr John Middleton, Vice President, UK Faculty of Public Health; Honorary Reader in Public Health, Birmingham University, UK

Dr Premila Webster, Head of School of Public Health at Health Education Thames Valley; Academic Registrar, UK Faculty of Public Health

Public health specialty registrars Helen Asquith, Beth Bennett-Britton, Lucy Douglas-Pannett, Emma Fletcher, Shamil Haroon, Sue Matthews, Susanna Mills, David Roberts, and Gemma Ward, for contributing to the Part B tips.

Health Education England (Thames Valley and West Midlands) for supporting Adam D M Briggs, Rob F Cooper and Paul A Fisher to pursue this project.

Our publishers for their support and understanding throughout the process of producing this book.

Finally, we and the publishers have attempted to seek permission from and to acknowledge all those whose work we used in compiling this book. If, however, we have unwittingly omitted any acknowledgements, then we apologise for this and please contact the Taylor & Francis Group.

Contributors

Angela Baker
Deputy Director
Public Health England South East
Public Health England
Chilton, Oxfordshire, United Kingdom

Adam D M Briggs
Wellcome Trust Research Training Fellow
Nuffield Department of Population Health
University of Oxford
Oxford, United Kingdom
and
Honorary Specialty Registrar in Public Health
Oxford University Hospitals NHS Trust
Oxford, United Kingdom

Christopher Chiswell
Consultant in Public Health
Birmingham Children's Hospital NHS Trust
Birmingham, United Kingdom

Rob F Cooper
Associate Postgraduate Dean and Head of School of Public Health
Health Education England (West Midlands)
Birmingham, United Kingdom
and
Honorary Senior Clinical Lecturer
University of Birmingham
Birmingham, United Kingdom

Paul A Fisher
Research Fellow in Public Health
School of Health and Population Sciences
University of Birmingham
Birmingham, United Kingdom

Rachael Leslie
Public Health Acting Consultant (Health Improvement)
Warwickshire County Council
Warwick, United Kingdom

Jill Meara
Director of Centre for Radiation Chemical and Environmental Hazards (CRCE)
Public Health England
Chilton, Oxfordshire, United Kingdom

Val Messenger
Deputy Director of Public Health
Oxfordshire County Council
Oxford, United Kingdom

Chris Packham
Associate Medical Director
Nottinghamshire Healthcare NHS Trust
and
Honorary Professor of Public Health Practice
University of Nottingham
Nottingham, United Kingdom
and
Chair of Examiners
OSPHE/Part B examination
Faculty of Public Health
United Kingdom

Nigel Smith
Tobacco Control, Physical Activity
and Sustainability
Public Health England Centre West Midlands
Birmingham, United Kingdom

Adam Turner
Leadership OD and Talent Programme Lead
Health Education England (West Midlands)
Birmingham, United Kingdom

Introduction

Practising public health is a unique opportunity to engage individuals, communities, organisations and populations to improve health and protect against disease. The purpose of this textbook is to help you to maximise your impact in the field and truly make a difference.

Public Health has been defined as 'The science and art of preventing disease, prolonging life and promoting health through the organised efforts of society' (Acheson, 1988); putting public health theory into practice sits at the interface between these two poles of the intellectual spectrum. This book aims to provide those either working in or preparing to work in public health with an appropriate skill set to maximise the impact of their day-to-day interactions. It is written for people with some prior experience of working in public health and takes a step-by-step approach through the specific challenges faced in health promotion, health protection, healthcare public health, and leadership and change management. Interspersed throughout each chapter are tips on practising public health as well as exercises to help put these tips into practice, explaining how to take the knowledge of public health theory and refine it to improve the health of populations.

Each chapter is broken down into an introduction, an overview of any relevant theory, and then detail on how to apply the theory to real-world scenarios. You will find frameworks, tips, examples and challenges throughout to illustrate appropriate communication skills, listening skills, information assimilation, reasoning and analytical skills, how to make appropriate public health judgements in given situations and how to handle uncertainty and conflict. The aim is for you to be able to use these examples and apply them to your own workplace. In order to support this, the glossary includes not only definitions of technical terms but also communication examples to translate complex public health concepts into lay language. Although the book is written for public health professionals with some prior knowledge and experience of public health, if you need a refresher in any topic, the pre-reading suggestions at the beginning of each chapter will help bring you up to speed with the underlying theory. 'Further Reading' at the end of each chapter as well as the reference list at the end of the book will direct you to further information.

The skills outlined above are tested by the UK Membership of the Faculty of Public Health (MFPH) of the Royal College of Physicians Part B exam, otherwise known as the Objective Structured Public Health Examination (OSPHE), are competency requirements for UK public health specialty registrars and form part of standards required for the UK Public Health Register or the public health designation of being on the General Medical Council specialist register in the UK. In the OSPHE the same five competences are tested independently at each of the six stations and this makes the overall assessment objective and a reliable measure of competency (Davison et al., 2010). Similar requirements are needed to be placed on the equivalent specialist registers in other countries. The online videos, along with the examination packs and examiners' feedback, offer the unique opportunity for prospective OSPHE candidates to observe and mark a scenario, and then to see how their marking compares to marks awarded by experienced OSPHE examiners. Tips from previously successful candidates can be found in Chapter 5.

The OSPHE seeks to identify individuals who have an appreciation of, and ability to demonstrate, the skills and attitudes relating to everyday public health issues – putting the theory into practice. These are skills and attitudes required of all professionals working in public health, and therefore the videos and examiners' comments will also be a key guide to those working in public health but not necessarily with any intention of sitting the OSPHE.

Working in public health is difficult, with a wide range of challenges that need to be overcome. However, the rewards can be great with the potential to make meaningful improvements to the health of populations and individuals. We hope that this book provides the support and guidance needed to maximise your impact in the field.

List of acronyms

AAA	Abdominal aortic aneurysm
ALSs	Action learning sets
ARR	Absolute risk reduction
BAC	Bronchioloalveolar carcinoma
BCG	Bacillus Calmette-Guérin (vaccine against tuberculosis)
BMJ	British Medical Journal
CBRN	Chemical, biological, radiological or nuclear [events]
CI	Confidence interval
CIN	Cervical intraepithelial neoplasia
DPH	Director of Public Health
DRGs	Diagnostic-related groups
DSR	Directly standardised rate
EOC	Emergency operation centre
EPPR	Emergency prevention preparedness and response
FPH	Faculty of Public Health
GDP	Gross domestic product
GMC	General Medical Council
GP	General practitioner
HIA	Health impact assessment
HPA	Health Protection Agency
HPV	Human papilloma virus
HRGs	Healthcare resource groups
ICD	Implantable cardiac defibrillator
ICER	Incremental cost-effectiveness ratio
JCVI	Joint Committee on Vaccines and Immunisations
LA	Local authority
LR	Likelihood ratio
MBTI	Myers-Briggs type indicator
MECC	Making every contact count
MFPH	Membership of the Faculty of Public Health
MP	Member of Parliament
MSF	Multi-source feedback (360 degree feedback)
NHS	UK National Health Service
NICE	National Institute for Health and Care Excellence
NNT	Number needed to treat
NPV	Negative predictive value
NSCLC	Non-small cell lung cancer
OR	Odds ratio
OSPHE	Objective Structured Public Health Examination
PACTS	Parliamentary Advisory Council for Transport Safety
PALS	Patient advisory and liaison service
PCO	Primary care organisation
PCT	Primary care trust
PDP	Personal development plan
PDSA	Plan, do, study, act
PESTLE	Political, economic, socio-cultural, technological, legal, environmental
PHE	Public Health England
PHSE	Personal health and social education
PHSKF	UK Public Health Skills and Knowledge Framework
PPE	Personal protective equipment
PPP	Purchasing power parities
PPV	Positive predictive value

PSA	Prostate-specific antigen
QALY	Quality-adjusted life year
ROI	Return on investment
RR	Relative risk
RRR	Relative risk reduction
SARS	Severe acute respiratory syndrome
SMART objectives	Specific, measurable, attainable, relevant and time-bound objectives
SSI	Slower speeds initiative
STAC	Scientific and Technical Advisory Cell
SWOT	Strengths, weaknesses, opportunities and threats
TB	Tuberculosis
UKPHR	UK Public Health Register
USD	U.S. dollar
WHO	World Health Organisation

List of videos and practising public health tips

Scenario	Description	URL
Scenario 1	Infection Hazards of Human Cadavers	http://goo.gl/IleQ7N
Scenario 2	Land Contamination in a Residential Area	http://goo.gl/ubPL7y
Scenario 3	HPV Vaccine to Prevent Cervical Cancer	http://goo.gl/omN5tF
Scenario 4	Interview on Speed Cameras	http://goo.gl/83R0Hb
Scenario 5	Exceptional Funding Request	http://goo.gl/ICTj3M
Scenario 6	Breast Screening Uptake Rates	http://goo.gl/ANM1pH
Scenario 7	Emergency Hospital Admissions	http://goo.gl/Lgka1m
Scenario 8	Smoking Ban	http://goo.gl/Gbn7lz

Tip Number	Subject	Page
Chapter 1	**Health Protection**	
1.1	Managing a health protection scenario	3
1.2	Communicating proactively	4
1.3	Describing data	6
1.4	Focusing on the outcome	6
1.5	Communicating risk	8
1.6	Discussing communicable disease	9
1.7	Predicting questions	9
1.8	Discussing inequalities	11
1.9	Using illustrations	13
1.10	Dealing with individual cases	16
1.11	Using diagrams	16
1.12	Practising technical terms	16
1.13	Checking journalists' understanding	18
1.14	Using social media	19
1.15	Ending conversations	19
Chapter 2	**Health promotion**	
2.1	Commissioning services	33
2.2	Using behaviour change models	33
2.3	Triggers for interventions	34
2.4	Benchmarking performance	34
2.5	Different data sources	34
2.6	Clear proposals	38
2.7	Using three key messages	38
2.8	Non-verbal communication	39
2.9	Using the media	42
Chapter 3	**Healthcare public health**	
3.1	Working in and with healthcare organisations	46
3.2	Prioritisation	49
3.3	Critical appraisal of evidence	50
3.4	Seven Cs of data appraisal	52
3.5	Case-mix analysis	52
Chapter 4	**Leadership and change management**	
4.1	Leadership styles	71
4.2	Successful meetings	82
4.3	Providing context	83

1

Health protection

PAUL A FISHER AND NIGEL SMITH

Introduction	2
Skills required for effective communication	3
Setting the scene	3
Risk communication	7
How safe is 'safe enough'?	8
Outbreaks and incidents	8
Communicating the risk of clusters	12
Emergency prevention preparedness and response	13
Screening	14
Talking to the public	16
Dealing with the media	16
Social media	18
Further reading	19

PRE-READING

- A general introduction can be found in Section 2 of Lewis G, Sheringham J, Lopez Bernal J, and Crayford T, *Mastering Public Health: A Postgraduate Guide to Examinations and Revalidation*, 2nd ed., CRC Press, Boca Raton, FL, 2014.
- Infectious disease (especially tuberculosis), contaminated land (specifically lead) and radiation (particularly radon) – Public Health England (PHE) has a Topics A–Z page (https://www.gov.uk/health-protection/infectious-diseases).
- Prostate cancer screening (used as an example in this section) – National Health Service (NHS) Cancer Screening Programmes are part of Public Health England, and NHS England has produced the national delivery framework for screening (http://www.cancerscreening.nhs.uk).
- Emergency prevention preparedness and response (EPPR) arrangements – NHS England has produced the strategic national framework for England (http://www.england.nhs.uk/ourwork/eprr/).
- In addition, wider reading of the PHE site (https://www.gov.uk/government/organisations/public-health-england) will provide background information on a broad range of health protection issues.

INTRODUCTION

Health protection is one of the three pillars of public health (alongside health promotion and healthcare public health) and covers a wide area including communicable disease, immunisation, screening, emergency prevention preparedness and response (EPPR) as well as environmental concerns including chemical and radiation issues.

Good communication skills are paramount to managing all the scenarios listed above. This is particularly true when there is a requirement, as there often is, to work with external stakeholders such as the public, media and other agencies. Possible situations that health protection professionals may be called upon to deal with and demonstrate effective communication skills in include managing incidents and outbreaks, surveillance, evaluating and explaining the need for immunisation, screening, cluster investigations and major disasters.

While dealing with these scenarios, a public health professional may need to communicate in multiple ways via several mediums to a variety of stakeholders. It is therefore important that public health professionals are well versed on the challenges of working:

- With limited information in rapidly developing situations
- In multi-agency scenarios incorporating multiple cultures and ways of doing things
- With the public including pressure groups
- With traditional media (newspapers, radio and TV)
- With social media (Twitter, Facebook, etc.)

Health protection issues may be acute (short-term incidents over a day or two, for example, a food poisoning outbreak at a wedding or a typical factory fire) or chronic (longer-term incidents, for example, tyre fires that can last for months or contaminated land issues where people may have been exposed for decades), both of which can present significant communication challenges for professionals. In acute settings the information available can change rapidly and there is often a great deal of uncertainty as the situation develops. In chronic situations the need for effective communication may increase over time, and there may be well-informed and well-organised protest groups involved who are able to rally and influence public concerns as well as local (and sometimes national) political debate. Regardless of whether these concerns are justified or not, it is important that public-facing organisations manage concerns well, ensure that information is based on the best known evidence and deliver it in a manner appropriate to the situation.

For example, during the 2009 H1N1 influenza pandemic, public health professionals were faced with a constantly changing scenario which made communicating consistent messages very challenging, especially to an extremely concerned and speculative public audience. As the pandemic unfolded, the types and methods of data being collected changed a number of times, making it very difficult to deliver consistent messages about numbers of cases to the media and public. Communicating effectively in these situations is paramount if health protection professionals are to maintain public trust.

There are often broadly similar elements in the response to health protection issues. Usually there is a need to gather and confirm information, assess the risk (often using a source-pathway-receptor model as described in detail in Section 'Outbreaks and Incidents'), identify control measures, communicate to stakeholders (including members of the public and the media) and monitor the situation. This response is frequently undertaken within a formal multi-agency response structure, and there is usually an organisation identified to lead on communication, to ensure that the correct message is being delivered.

This chapter discusses the relevant communication skills required for working as a public health professional focusing on how to set the scene, risk communication, dealing with outbreaks, and screening, and finishes off with a 'Social Media' section on dealing with the media. We have chosen two example scenarios to illustrate the techniques that can be utilised to effectively communicate health protection information:

1. Communicating to the media regarding communicable disease (tuberculosis [TB]), environmental (lead) contamination and radiation (radon) incidents

2. Communicating to a local politician about the pros and cons of a prostate cancer screening programme

Practising public health tip 1.1 Managing a health protection scenario: Typically when managing a health protection scenario, the following skills are tested:

- The need to provide data in a meaningful way
- The interpretation of complex and often incomplete data
- Dealing with uncertainty
- The public health relevance of the information or the situation that needs to be understood and conveyed
- The next steps in dealing with the situation

SKILLS REQUIRED FOR EFFECTIVE COMMUNICATION

A range of skills is required to communicate public health issues effectively. More specifically, health protection professionals need to be mindful of the following when communicating an important public health message:

Clarity: Be sure what you convey is clear. Good clear delivery of messages is important in both verbal and non-verbal communication. While often daunting, it is useful to practise delivering messages with a friend or colleague who will provide feedback on pace, content and clarity. It is essential to limit the use of medical and statistical phrases when communicating to non-health professionals, and clearly explain any jargon used (see Glossary).

Consistency and confidence: Provide a steady narrative. Public health professionals are often put into situations where all the information may not be available or the situation changes. However, a stable, confident message must be delivered throughout, with clear justification of any changes to this message over time.

Transparency: Tell people what you can. While it may not always be prudent to share every detail (for example, where information is not available or too much information would dilute the message we are trying to convey), it is important that we do not appear to be hiding information or seem dishonest.

Accuracy: Focus on the knowns, not the unknowns. Situations vary and there may be many unknowns. Therefore it isn't always possible to provide specific details. However, it is important that the information we do give is as accurate as possible and that we try not to speculate. For example, if the evidence is the best or most recent, then we have to say that.

Timeliness: Provide information when it is required. Knowing when to listen and when to deliver important messages is an art form in itself. If faced with an upset parent, we cannot bombard them with information and think our job is done; we need to listen and then respond, adjusting our tone to the situation.

Be proactive: Don't wait for media interest before communicating on an issue. When an issue needs to be communicated in the interest of public health or to allay public fears, it is easier to control the situation by timely proactive messages in the first place than reacting to stories after they have been produced. The timeliness of these proactive messages is especially important as information can be communicated quickly (and possibly twisted via the wrong sources).

SETTING THE SCENE

One of the foundations of good communication is the ability to understand the viewpoint of the person you are having the conversation with. This allows you to understand why they are saying certain things, what they want to hear from you and how you need to respond.

Thinking through the following four questions will help you to achieve a positive outcome in a communication scenario:

Question 1 What am I trying to say and why?
Question 2 Who am I saying it to?
Question 3 What is the best way to communicate the message?
Question 4 What might their reaction be to what I'm saying?

These four questions will be covered in detail below.

Question 1 What am I trying to say and why?

There may be certain information that needs to be relayed; however, it is important to keep in mind the purpose of the conversation. For example, are you:

- Trying to reassure?
- Asserting control?
- Providing information?
- Attempting to change someone's behaviour?
- Negotiating – trying to agree or change an arrangement or contract?
- Trying to change someone's opinion?

Practising public health tip 1.2
Communicating proactively: Regardless of the situation you should try to be as helpful as possible. Public health professionals can often take a defensive approach – the less you say, the less the chance of making a mistake – but appearing to be evasive or unhelpful can make the situation worse. A more proactive, positive approach is the most likely tactic to contribute to successful communication.

Question 2 Who am I saying it to?

The amount of detail required, the language used, the degree of emotional intelligence (e.g. empathy) needed and what a successful outcome to the conversation would look like all depend on who you are speaking to and what their concerns are.

EXERCISE 1.1

Think about conversations with (1) media, (2) the public, (3) other professionals and (4) politicians. What particular communication challenges might arise with these different groups and how would you know if your tactic to overcome these issues had been successful?

Typical situations and key issues to consider are summarised in Table 1.1.

During a long-term chronic incident a communication strategy may need to be developed (or for common events one could already be in place). These will often have identified key people who need to be kept informed of the situation and will detail how much resource should be given to each stakeholder dependent on their likely interest in the incident and their power to influence or assist. This will help ensure efforts are targeted efficiently and effectively. Knowing which quadrant in the communication grid a stakeholder belongs to will also help tailor the message. Table 1.2 demonstrates an example of what could be produced by a local government authority for use during a seasonal flu pandemic (Figure 1.3 shows a variation on a communication grid for analysing stakeholders).

Question 3 What is the best way to communicate the message?

The most important element of clear communication is to have a logical structure. To assist the public health professional there are a number of frameworks available, for example:

- Incident management
  - Say what has happened/is happening at the moment
  - Say what is being done – assert reassurance and that things are under control (or not)
  - Say what people can do (e.g. self-help)
- Talking to the media: ABC
  - **A**nswer the question/issue
  - **B**ridge conversation to the public health message
  - **C**ommunicate the public health message
- Talking to the media: three key messages
  - Before the interview, think of your three key messages you want to get across and use every opportunity to repeat them during the interview
- Talking to the public when sympathy is required, e.g. following a death: 3Rs
  - **R**egret (express regret for an event that has happened)
  - **R**eason (state why it happened)

Table 1.1 Key issues to consider when speaking to different stakeholders

Stakeholder	Possible situations	Key considerations	What success would look like
Public	Concern about relatives Anger over lack of perceived action Fear of possible threats to health and safety (short term and long term) Death of a loved one	An appropriate emotional response, e.g. sympathy in the event of a death Showing empathy and understanding, e.g. when talking about immunisation in respect of a loved one As public health professionals we must always be respectful, regardless of public reaction	Member of the public is reassured Extreme reactions may be tempered if the individual(s) feel as though you are treating them with respect
Media	Trying to find someone to blame Requiring information to provide to the public Wanting a 'good news' story Wanting to be the first to publish	Do not try to blame other organisations or communicate information that could potentially harm their reputations May not be able to share information about suspected sources due to the need to maintain confidentiality Information may not be as up to date or as accurate as they might want Be proactive, open and transparent	Media provide useful public health messages especially during emergency situations, e.g. outbreaks Media are willing to work with you, not against you
Other professionals (e.g. environmental health officer)	Need to decide what needs to be done and which organisation will be responsible for actions	Statutory responsibilities of the agencies	Agreement between organisations and well-defined actions assigned to the correct agency
Politician (e.g. councillor)	Wanting certain action to resolve an issue Focused primarily on the interests of their constituents	Often there are limitations to what can be done (financial, scientific, legal, political and statutory)	Agreed action that satisfies stakeholders and does not compromise or dilute the public health message

- **R**emedy/**r**esponse (say what is going to be done about it)
- Describing data
  - **1** – Describe the type of data (e.g. graph of influenza rates)
  - **2** – Describe what it shows (e.g. an increase every winter)
  - **3** – Describe the key features (e.g. increase this winter is an order of magnitude higher than other winters displayed)
  - **4** – Outline possible reasons (e.g. this could be due to a new strain of influenza)

Table 1.2 Example of communication grid to ensure efficient use of resources

Power	Level of interest	
	Low	**High**
Low	**A – Minimal effort** Optometrists	**B – Keep informed** Practice staff Dentists Users of public transport Carers Council staff Independent providers
High	**C – Keep satisfied** Schoolchildren Local businesses Local community/patient/public groups	**D – Key players** Schoolteachers Parents Primary care: GPs, practice staff, pharmacists National and regional health organisations Local media Elected members

Practising public health tip 1.3 Describing data: When describing data the following issues should be considered:

- Limitations of data.
- Are patterns true or an artefact (coding or reporting error, introduction of screening programme, change in practice, change in denominator)?
- Chance – small numbers – look for significant difference (confidence intervals), trends.
- Confounding factors – age, gender, case mix, deprivation, ethnicity – need to standardise, adjust.
- Bias – data collection, randomisation, intention to treat.
- Note: When using statistical terms do not assume that the person you are communicating to understands what you mean; you may need to explain it in plain terms (see Glossary).

Question 4 What might their reaction be to what I'm saying?

It is essential that before you communicate any information to stakeholders, you consider first how they might react to it. Therefore you need to consider:

- Who it is being said to
- The time at which it is said
- The tone in which it is said

Practising public health tip 1.4 Focusing on the outcome: It is important to understand the answer to Question 1 early on in any conversation to understand what focus you need to give and what is the successful target for the exchange. For instance, if it is reassurance, you may want to focus on reframing the risk in common terms (for example, comparing emissions from a fire to those typical for bonfire night). If it is about providing information, ensure you have been as comprehensive as possible, check understanding and ensure your language is suitable for the stakeholder you are talking to. Part of this answer may only become apparent during the exchange so you need to be ready to respond to new directions taken.

Try to ensure you know the answer to Question 2 beforehand, and if not, ask as soon as possible. For Question 3, remember that different people process information differently and just because a strategy has worked in the past it does not mean it will again. The key tactic is ordering information so you can build up a story and, most importantly, gauge what level of existing understanding there is (if you are unclear, then feel free to check: 'Are you following this'? 'Ask me if you want me to explain any terms', 'Please stop me at any point if you don't understand').

The answer to Question 4 will usually only be apparent during the conversation and you will have to alter your style as appropriate (for example, trying to defuse the situation and show empathy if the individual is angry).

Public health professionals can focus on the active skill of speaking over the passive skill of listening (which is often more important). This is particularly true in exam situations (such as the Part B exam) where understanding of the scenario is only covered in part in the exam paperwork provided and therefore carefully listening to the examiner is key to understand:

- How to respond effectively
- When you are being helped
- When further information is being sought

What is most important is that you succinctly answer the questions, deliver your key messages and respond to queries. Do not feel you have to fill as much of the allocated time as possible with your own voice.

Finally, understanding body language (both your own and that of your audience) is important and can help professionals understand the situation more clearly and respond more appropriately. For example, if the person is upset, you need to utilise this information to decide upon the best way to proceed – it might simply be to first let them speak and you listen sympathetically (making sure your own body language reflects this), before responding appropriately.

RISK COMMUNICATION

Risk is a key element of any health protection scenario. This can be difficult to explain to stakeholders for a number of reasons:

- Levels of uncertainty about the situation.
- Language used to describe risk by professionals can involve a lot of jargon. Also many words mean different things to different organisations, for example, the difference between a hazard and a risk.
- There can be a large difference between the understanding of risk within the public health profession and the perception of risk among the general public, politicians and other professionals.

Health protection messages generally aim to inform, reassure or warn. Sometimes the message given will involve all three, for example, telling the public about a chemical fire that is producing toxic emissions (warning the public of danger) and advising people to stay indoors, keeping doors and windows closed (informing them of the action to take to reduce the risk), while stressing this is a precautionary approach and there are unlikely to be any long-term impacts on health (reassuring).

How you state a risk will influence how it is understood, so it is important to choose the right way that suits the situation. For example, telling someone that a procedure 'has a 90% survival rate' will be viewed as far more promising than if they are told that 'there is a 10% mortality rate' even though both statements are describing the same statistic.

EXERCISE 1.2

What elements of a hazard might increase the risk perception of the general public?

Regardless of the size of the risk, it is more likely to be unacceptable to the public if it is:

- Involuntary rather than voluntary – people may underestimate the risk of activities they choose (e.g. smoking, skiing) and overestimate risks that are imposed on them (e.g. air pollution, chemicals in the food chain).

- Novel rather than longstanding – people may overplay the risk of new diseases such as severe acute respiratory syndrome (SARS; a respiratory disease caused by the SARS coronavirus) and underestimate the risk of existing diseases like seasonal flu.
- Man-made rather than natural – for example, if a chemical is found naturally (e.g. arsenic), the risk is likely to be more acceptable than an equally dangerous chemical that is produced in a laboratory.
- Relating to children rather than adults – issues surrounding children can be more emotive than those concerning adults and therefore great care must be taken, for example, using the right tone to prevent panic.
- A disease associated with dread – such as cancer or dementia rather than, for example, heart disease. Interestingly, this can change over time; TB used to be the disease of dread in the nineteenth century in the UK, but in the twenty-first century it is cancer in the under 65s and dementia in the over 65 population.

Therefore the health protection professional can try to identify the sort of response they are likely to receive when giving public health messages based upon the type of risk involved.

HOW SAFE IS 'SAFE ENOUGH'?

In encounters public health professionals will often have to deal with the concept as to whether or not something or some situation can be described as 'safe'. Stakeholders often want to be reassured that there is no risk, but unfortunately this is never absolutely the case, as the sixteenth-century physician Paracelsus stated, 'The dose makes the poison' – even water can be fatal if you drink enough. Common approaches to tackling this problem are:

- Referring to the legal requirements (such as soil guideline values for contaminated land)
- Stating there is no evidence of harm (for example, not picked up by current surveillance systems)
- Relating the risk to other common risks that people can relate to (for instance, small cancer risks to natural rare events like being struck by lightning)

Practising public health tip 1.5
Communicating risk: When discussing what is safe, have a good understanding of how a certain risk relates to common risks:

- Minimal risk – killed by lightning: 1 in 10 million
- Very low risk – death by rail crash: 1 in 1 million
- Low risk – death by murder: 1 in 100,000
- Moderate risk – death by road traffic accident in a year: 1 in 10,000
- High risk – death by all causes before the age of 40: 1 in 1000

Understanding where the risk lies on this continuum (true risk) and where the stakeholder thinks the risk lies (risk perception) will help you frame your communication around what is safe.

OUTBREAKS AND INCIDENTS

EXERCISE 1.3

What are the key questions you would want answered when you are contacted about an incident or outbreak?

When gathering information about an incident, the following questions typically need to be answered:

1. **Who?**
   Who has contacted you? Who is involved? Are there any casualties (number killed, hospitalised, infected and decontaminated)? Are there any vulnerable groups? What other agencies are involved and what are the command and control arrangements? Who is talking about the incident (e.g. traditional media, people on social media, etc.)?
2. **What?**
   What has happened? What is the organism, chemical, type of radiation involved? What are the symptoms? What are the weather conditions? What is our or my involvement? What advice (shelter, evacuation, decontamination) has already been given? What has been said to the media?

Practising public health tip 1.6 Discussing communicable disease: When discussing communicable disease situations with colleagues and stakeholders, make sure you are clear about the key elements of the disease, for example:

- Method of transmission (e.g. airborne)
- Incubation period
- Period of communicability
- Symptoms
- Severity of the disease
- Treatment of the disease
- Measures to prevent the spread of disease

3. **Where?**
   Where is the incident? Where is the control centre? Where is the source? Is it likely to spread anywhere (e.g. a plume of chemicals from a fire)?
4. **When?**
   When did the incident occur? When were you contacted? When is the next meeting? When do decisions need to be made? How long is the incident likely to last? When will control measures be in place?
5. **Why?**
   Why is this a public health issue?
6. **How?**
   How will we be able to measure the severity of the problem? How will the situation be resolved?

Being able to answer these questions will be of great benefit to successfully communicating health protection issues. As well as being the key questions that we as public health professionals need to ask, they are also the questions that all stakeholders, especially the media, will want to know the answers to.

Furthermore, it is important to have a good general knowledge of the topic (though with novel scenarios this will be less easy) so you can speak confidently about the subject and answer any questions that might come up. Finally, it is useful to have an understanding of what success looks like – what is the aim of communication in your situation? For example, the goal could be reassurance, the provision of information or influencing behaviour via the provision of key public health messages (it is often useful to choose and then focus on three key messages).

Practising public health tip 1.7 Predicting questions: If you have time before going into a meeting with a colleague or member of the media to discuss a communicable disease situation, think about the types of questions that might come up and prepare some answers. Typical questions could be:

- What are the risks to the local community?
- Is it serious?
- What have you done/are you doing/will you be doing next?
- Who is responsible?
- Who might object, try to apportion blame, etc. – i.e. what are the potential negative issues that could arise and from where could they be raised (e.g. pressure groups, media, etc.)?
- What will my response be?

To illustrate the points above, consider the following three scenarios and think about what you might need to know and what you can communicate, for example, to a journalist:

1. You have recently been notified of a case of TB in a school (example of an acute incident).
2. Sampling has identified high levels of heavy metal contamination in soil at residential properties (example of a chronic incident).
3. A local government authority and PHE are setting up a system of monitoring radon levels in residential properties to identify ones that would benefit from remediation (example of a measure to reduce risk/exposure).

EXERCISE 1.4

For these three situations consider:

- What are the questions you would want answers to?
- What information would you be expected to know as a health protection professional?
- What organisations would be involved?
- What communication challenges might there be?
- What public health messages would you want to provide?

Table 1.3 Issues to consider in health protection incidents

	TB outbreak at school	Residential properties on contaminated land	Radon in residential properties
Who?	One child infected, children and staff in class at risk	No one identified as affected, all residents at potential risk	1000 deaths per year in UK, whole population at risk (particularly smokers, those in high radon areas, households with basements)
What?	TB	Heavy metals, cancer and neurological disease	Radon, lung cancer
Where?	School, classroom	Gardens	Houses
When?	First symptoms, confirmed, school notified, parents notified, testing to occur, results provided	Land first contaminated, exposure over period since properties built, testing to occur, results	Chronic issue, would have been a problem from when the properties were first built
Why?	There is a possible risk to children and staff who have been in prolonged contact in a confined space	Possible risk to residents of long-term exposure	Risk to population of lung cancer
How?	All children in class to be given a blood test to see if they have TB	Series of soil samples taken	Testing of properties, remediation
Key knowledge and skills	Natural history of TB Outbreak investigation Risk communication	Health impacts of heavy metal Risk communication	Health effects of radon Risk communication
Other stakeholders	School management National, regional and local health professionals (public health, providers and commissioners) Local authority (LA) Parents Media	Developers Environmental organisations Local health protection teams National and regional chemical and environmental experts LA – contaminated land Residents Media	Local health protection teams National and regional chemical and environmental experts LA – housing Residents Media
Potential issues	Worried well/is my child at risk? Why aren't children/infants routinely given BCG? Cultural issues/blame	Worried well Fear of financial loss Who's to blame? LA? Private developer?	Worried well Who's to blame? LA? Private developer?
Public health messages	Risk is low Testing will identify those with disease Treatment available What the symptoms are What to do if you are concerned	Risk is low Testing will identify if remediation is required What the symptoms are What to do if you have symptoms	Risk may be high, particularly if you are a smoker in a high radon area How to get testing kit Problem is treatable (remediation with sump and fan)

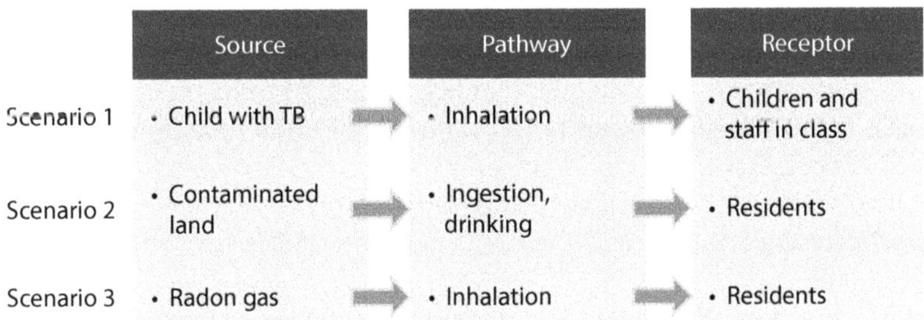

Figure 1.1 The source-pathway-receptor model.

Example responses to the questions that need to be answered for these three scenarios have been summarised in Table 1.3.

To answer questions about the severity of a situation, a risk assessment needs to be undertaken. A systematic way of approaching this is the source-pathway-receptor model. To understand the risk, we need to know what the problem is, who could be affected and how the issue could travel to a given individual. How this model would be utilised in the three examples above can be seen in Figure 1.1.

Understanding this model is important for health protection communication, as removing one of these elements is often the basis for putting control measures in place. For example, in Figure 1.1 we could remove the source in scenario 1 (removing the child with TB from the class while they are being treated), remove the pathway in scenario 2 (asking people to wash any vegetables they are growing, concrete over the land) or remove the receptors in scenario 3 (residents moved to temporary accommodation while remediation is carried out).

Practising public health tip 1.8 Discussing inequalities: With incidents where there are often elements of health or environmental inequalities, you may be asked to describe who the vulnerable groups are or how environmental inequalities can be reduced (for example, which areas should be prioritised for remediation given a limited budget).

For outbreaks there is a set of steps for a typical investigation as detailed in Box 1.1. Communication can be critical at each stage, and improving communication is the most frequent recommendation made during debriefs. During a high-profile investigation it will be important to keep stakeholders, including the media and general public, abreast of what stage an investigation is at.

BOX 1.1: Twelve stages of outbreak investigation

1. Establish that a problem exists.
2. Confirm the diagnosis – case definition (clinical or laboratory confirmed).
3. Outline the immediate control measures – utilising the source (control), pathway (interrupt transmission), receptor (protect those at risk) model.
4. List the case findings – cases initially notified are often only a small proportion of existing cases. Further cases found through notifications, laboratory results, NHS usage (calls to NHS 111, general practitioner [GP] attendance, hospital emergency department, hospital inpatients and outpatients), occupational health departments, school absenteeism, appeals through local and national media and screening programmes.
5. Collect data – ideally face-to-face using a semi-structured questionnaire.

6. Describe epidemiology – cases described by time, person and place.
7. Generate hypothesis– what is the source? What is the route of transmission?
8. Test hypothesis – microbiological/environmental investigation or epidemiological study (case control study or cohort).
9. List further control measures – surveillance and updating of the epidemic curve to allow outbreak to be declared over.
10. Declare incident over.
11. Conduct wash-up, hot debrief (a few days later) and cold debrief (a few weeks later).
12. Write incident report.

COMMUNICATING THE RISK OF CLUSTERS

Patterns can always be found in the distribution of disease due to natural variation. Often public concern with a cluster of disease is whether the particular pattern is due to increased risk from a specific source, often a current or historic industrial facility or a landfill site.

The first issue that needs to be communicated is that, in a given area, there are going to be more cases of disease if there are greater numbers of people (for example, there will be clusters around towns and villages) or there are more people with risk factors (for example, clusters of cancer around retirement villages) so numbers have to be converted into age-standardised rates to take account of this.

However, once standardisation has been applied, it would still not be expected that disease is perfectly evenly spaced (as illustrated in Figure 1.2 where each triangle is a case of disease), although this may be the understanding among non-epidemiologists. Just as there are natural variations in, for example, weather patterns, we would expect there to be natural variations in disease distribution even if all relevant factors were standardised; natural clusters are likely to form randomly (as shown in Figure 1.3), with nothing to do with any increased risk associated with that area.

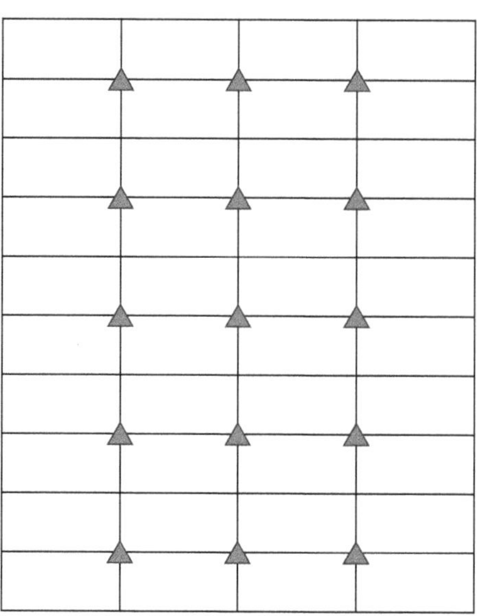

Figure 1.2 Map showing evenly spaced cases of disease.

The final effect is often referred to as the Texas sharpshooter effect. If bullets were fired at a wall and then the target were drawn around where they centred, anyone could be made to look like a magnificent shot. With similar logic, if a potential source (the star in Figure 1.4), such as an industrial site, is identified in the centre of a cluster, then the pattern of disease would look incriminating. However, this may be less to do with a relationship of increasing risk for people living closer to a site than the fact that the site was chosen as it was in the middle of a cluster of disease.

Communicating the science behind cluster investigations can be an example of when a diagram can speak a thousand words. A simple map, such as the ones shown in Figures 1.2 through 1.4, can be extremely useful in communicating this risk to members of the public.

It also illustrates the complexity of communicating some of these issues to laypeople and highlights the need to explain via a series of simple steps, checking comprehension at each stage, rather than trying to get people to understand the real (rather than perceived) risk in one go.

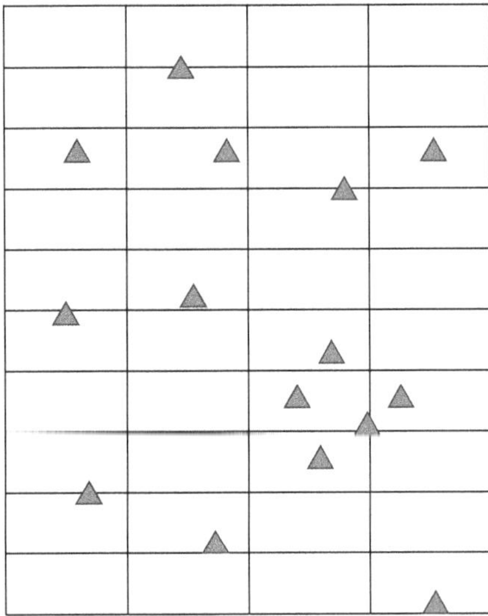

Figure 1.3 Map showing random pattern of cases of disease.

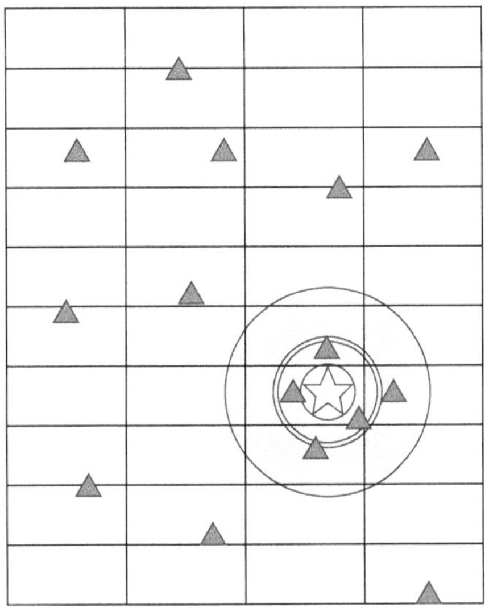

Figure 1.4 Map showing a potential cluster of cases (circles) with a central source (star).

Practising public health tip 1.9 Using illustrations: Do not be afraid to sketch out a quick diagram if you think it will help illustrate a point. Furthermore, having a diagram and putting it on the table between you and the person you are talking to naturally brings the two people together, giving a focal point for the discussion.

EMERGENCY PREVENTION PREPAREDNESS AND RESPONSE

It is important to understand the most up-to-date EPPR structures (at the time of writing the latest structures in England are detailed in NHS England guidance). Knowledge of these structures will enable professionals to clearly explain the wider response required to stakeholders and also ensure they are informing all the other relevant stakeholders.

Public health professionals may be involved in a variety of emergency situations including fires posing a threat to the public, as well as rarer mass casualty situations due to chemical, biological, radiological or nuclear (CBRN) events. CBRN emergencies can occur as a result of industrial disasters, occupational exposures, natural catastrophes, warfare or acts of terrorism.

There are regular training sessions for people who are likely to take up specific roles in dealing with emergencies, for example, as part of an emergency operation centre (EOC) or a Scientific and Technical Advisory Cell (STAC). The EOC is a central command and control facility responsible for collecting, gathering and analysing data in order to form a strategic overview of the disaster and make operational decisions. The STAC provides strategic command with advice on issues such as the impact of disasters on the health of the population and environmental protection as well as sampling and monitoring of contaminants. Attending this type of training will help professionals understand how information should be communicated during the heat of an incident.

A working knowledge of the basic terminology used by the emergency services is essential for quickly understanding and keeping up with rapidly developing situations that are typical of emergencies. For instance, the central area with the spill, fire, leak, etc. is called the hot zone; any casualties will be taken to the warm zone for treatment or decontamination while the majority of personnel will be in the relative safety of the cold zone (Figure 1.5). If the contamination is airborne, the warm zone will be upwind of the hot zone.

One of the key decisions in these incidents is how and where to carry out decontamination. As

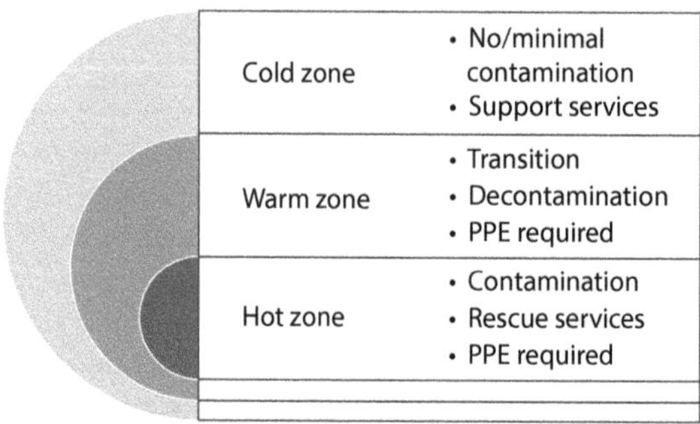

Figure 1.5 Zones at an incident. PPE, personal protective equipment.

much as possible, this should be carried out on site in the transition between the warm zone and the cold zone. This ensures decontamination occurs as soon as possible and also reduces the risk of ambulances becoming contaminated and put out of service at the time they are needed the most. Further decontamination at the hospital can often be carried out outside the building itself, so reducing the risk of contaminating critical parts of the hospital (e.g. the emergency department).

Giving instructions to members of the public during decontamination is one of the most difficult communication tasks health professionals can face due to the stress both sides may be under. It is, however, one of the most important, as clearly following instructions may significantly reduce the risk to the individual. Effective communication can significantly increase compliance, reduce anxiety and lower the risk of mass panic. Examples of poor communication include not explaining the need for decontamination (i.e. the health risk), not respecting a person's need for privacy and not being clear (for example, not using a loudhailer or not using simple language). Attending exercises to practise the communication skills specific to decontamination can be extremely useful so that during the heat of an incident clear communication becomes second nature.

Triage is a critical step in emergencies for categorising the casualties in accordance with medical care priorities. This could be done in the hot zone (may involve tagging people with different colours so those who will benefit the most from help get it quickest), warm zone (deciding on who needs to attend hospital) or at various stages at the hospital

Table 1.4 Different levels of incident command in England

Command level	Area of command	Location
Platinum	National	Cabinet Office Briefing Room
Gold	Strategic	Usually chaired by the police at a distant location
Silver	Tactical	Often in a command vehicle or police station close to the scene
Bronze	Operational	On scene in the cold zone

(for example, who needs to be admitted). Again, spending time and effort to communicate this process to the public will ensure a smoother procedure and calmer patients.

Another key discussion, and an important message that needs to be communicated to the public, is whether to give shelter or evacuation advice. If possible this will be informed by monitoring (either personal or fixed monitoring) and modelling (for example, simple maps showing wind direction, called chemical meteorology in England, or more detailed air pollution modelling). However, given the timescales, detailed monitoring and modelling are not always possible, and so a precautionary approach is often taken. This generally means shelter advice is given (go in, stay in, tune in) unless there is an explosion risk (in which case there will be a cordon that will need to be evacuated around the site) or the incident is particularly hazardous or is likely to last a long time, in which case evacuation advice may need to be given.

Table 1.4 illustrates how these decisions are made at varying levels of the command hierarchy.

SCREENING

Screening is an important process where a subpopulation or individual can be identified that has a disease or is at higher risk of developing a disease than the general population.

For example, cancer screening is a useful tool and can save lives, particularly when:

- The disease is common and causes significant mortality.
- There is a relatively harmless, sensitive screening test that can identify a cancer earlier than would be the case when waiting for symptoms to develop.
- There is a diagnostic test with a high specificity.
- There is an acceptable treatment available.

If these elements apply, then the cost-effectiveness of a screening programme could be considered.

However, the majority of cancers are not screened for on a population basis in the UK because these conditions are not met.

EXERCISE 1.5

Considering the four elements of cancer screening above, what would your arguments be for and against the introduction of a national prostate cancer screening programme?

For example, for prostate cancer:

- Although common, people are more likely to die with prostate cancer than from it as it is usually slow growing and not invasive.
- Tests result in a lot of false negatives and false positives.
- The diagnostic test can result in significant side effects (e.g. incontinence).
- There is a lack of evidence on treatment affecting the natural history of the disease.

To explain these relationships it is often easiest to talk about percentages. If 100 people over the age of 65 are screened, how many people will be helped? How many will have invasive treatment unnecessarily? How many will be told they have cancer who do not? Visuals have been developed to illustrate these risks to patients utilising a 10 × 10 grid of faces – smiley faces for those without the disease and sad faces for those with the disease. These can then be coloured differently or have a cross over them to illustrate false negatives, false positives and those who would likely die by other causes before the disease killed them.

For example, Figure 1.6 could be used to illustrate a screening test where (1) 6% of the population would benefit from the screening as their condition would be identified earlier and could be successfully treated, (2) 18% would be harmed by screening (for example, undergoing unnecessary treatment as they were false positives) and (3) the vast majority (76%) would not be affected (although their concern about the disease may have increased and there are opportunity costs to consider).

☺	☺	☺	☺	☺	☺	☹	☹	☹	☹
☹	☹	☹	☹	☹	☹	☹	☹	☹	☹
☹	☹	☹	☹	😐	😐	😐	😐	😐	😐
😐	😐	😐	😐	😐	😐	😐	😐	😐	😐
😐	😐	😐	😐	😐	😐	😐	😐	😐	😐
😐	😐	😐	😐	😐	😐	😐	😐	😐	😐
😐	😐	😐	😐	😐	😐	😐	😐	😐	😐
😐	😐	😐	😐	😐	😐	😐	😐	😐	😐
😐	😐	😐	😐	😐	😐	😐	😐	😐	😐
😐	😐	😐	😐	😐	😐	😐	😐	😐	😐

☺	People who benefit from screening
☹	People harmed by screening
😐	People not affected by screening

Figure 1.6 Communicating the risk of screening programmes.

Practising public health tip 1.10 Dealing with individual cases: When talking to lay people, individual cases will often be referenced (e.g. the person's relative or the individual themselves might have had a test that saved their life because a tumour was removed). In these situations it is often useful to try to turn the conversation, while acknowledging and not dismissing the individual's experience, around to the population level (e.g. if we take a 100 people with prostate cancer ...) rather than focusing on the individual case. This will hopefully enable a focus on the balance of benefits and harms where the whole population is considered.

Practising public health tip 1.11 Using diagrams: Consider using a simple diagram if you have enough preparation time, as this can be much easier and quicker than explaining something complex orally.

TALKING TO THE PUBLIC

It is important to use terms that the average member of the public will understand. This means using simpler language whenever possible, for example, 'a type of flu' rather than 'a H1N1 subtype of influenza A virus'. Ideally all jargon should be avoided, but when uncommon terms have to be used, they should be explained in simple terms (see the glossary).

Practising public health tip 1.12 Practising technical terms: Practise describing epidemiological terms (such as those in the glossary) with your friends and family.

DEALING WITH THE MEDIA

Getting conversations with the media right during an outbreak is essential as the media can be a key ally for health protection professionals; we need to make the most of every opportunity. Furthermore, you may be meeting the same journalist on a number of occasions during your role, so it is a good idea to build up a good relationship with them and present yourself as someone who can be approached for information. This can mean that journalists approach you first as an official source of information before looking for less reliable ones. During the 2009 influenza pandemic, public health sources became the first port of call for reliable information for journalists, which was of great benefit in ensuring that consistent scientific information dominated the media coverage.

Tips for dealing with the media include the following:

General

- Use your common sense. The majority of journalists will respect what you have to say and will not try to trip you up. However, it is always important that you remember that their goal is to write a story that will be read. Remember there is no such thing as 'off the record' and never say 'no comment'.

Preparation

- Establish as early as possible how and when you are going to communicate with the media. This is most relevant during major incidents and slow-burning incidents where multiple media interest is anticipated. For example, during a Legionnaires' outbreak in Hereford, England, in 2003, after initial press conferences, daily press statements were recorded on an answerphone message. During the 2009 influenza pandemic, NHS West Midlands issued twice daily press briefings by email containing news, events to date and self-help advice. While techniques like these cannot replace one-to-one contact with a journalist or answer specific questions, they reduce the impact on staff of constantly answering the same questions and they demonstrate that there is a plan in place.
- Understand in advance exactly what you are going to be asked to do, e.g. is it a radio interview? Will it be a telephone call or in the

studio? Will it be live or recorded? Live means that you cannot stop the interview if you make a mistake or are asked a question you do not have the answer to. However, it does allow the interviewee to communicate the messages they want to without fear of being edited.
- Ask in advance, where possible, what the questions are going to be so you can prepare – a good journalist will be happy to provide the questions as they want you be as relaxed and engaging as possible, as this makes for a polished performance and gives them an opportunity to develop their own line of questioning and enhances the development of local relationships.
- Develop your key messages before undertaking any interviews. Even if a journalist wants to interview you there and then, ask them for a few minutes to allow you to compose your messages. Develop a maximum of three or four messages that you want to convey during the interview and ensure you communicate them. If you are working with multiple agencies, then ensure that you have agreed on the messages prior to communicating with them. Try to make your messages as 'sticky' as possible, in other words memorable, easily digestible sound bites.

During

- Be honest – admit what you do not know. However, depending on the situation, be prepared to offer to follow the question up outside of the interview with someone who does know and then call the journalist to let them know the answer.
- Ensure your responses and body language are appropriate to the situation, for example, sympathetic and reassuring when individuals express concern. Avoid defensive or aggressive behaviour.
- Be positive where you can – often the risk of harm to the general public is extremely low. For example, in a Legionnaires' outbreak, explain the level of risk including that there is no person-to-person spread, who is most at risk, and that even if you are at risk there is help available, and then explain how to access that help.
- Focus on the action you are taking, e.g. developing a case definition, holding multi-agency meetings, testing samples at laboratories, working with national experts.
- Be prepared for hostile questioning. A journalist may believe that you are hiding information or that the actions you or other organisations have taken are insufficient or incorrect. Regardless of how the journalist behaves, you must ensure you remain calm, stick to your messages and don't get angry or upset.
- Stress the facts – only communicate what is known for certain.
- Only speak about topics your organisation has permitted you to talk about. Do not speak on behalf of other organisations unless permitted to do so.
- Give the wider context – for example, there might be a doubling of the risk of disease but as the baseline is 1 in 100,000, the absolute risk is minimal.
- Be firm but polite if you do not want to discuss a particular issue.
- Avoid discussions of money or cost savings – stress that your primary concern is the health of the population and you would like to focus on that.
- Avoid speculation.
- Avoid criticisms of other groups or individuals.
- There are often issues with poor communication during incidents so respond to criticism by focusing on how information flow can be improved in the future.
- Unless there is agreement with the individual or organisation prior to an interview, you must not share patient identifiable information or information about a company that is suspected of being responsible for an outbreak.

After

- Ask to see a draft copy of an article before it is published. Journalists will often be more than happy to accommodate these requests as you are basically providing a free proofreading service.

Practising public health tip 1.13 Checking journalists' understanding: When discussing with a journalist, the need to correct a misunderstanding of the data/situation can arise. Ensure that the journalist has a correct understanding of the situation and use the opportunity to provide information to the public (regardless of the questions the journalist is asking). You can then go on to communicating your public health messages.

SOCIAL MEDIA

Social media is a relatively new phenomenon in regard to communicating public health messages; however, it is becoming as influential as traditional media.

Social media constitutes many different platforms. It is generally accepted that the two that public health professionals are concerned with (at the time of writing) are Facebook and Twitter. However, the considerations that are discussed below can be applied to most platforms.

Despite ongoing hesitancy about using social media due to its immediacy and perceived lack of control, it cannot be ignored by health protection professionals as it has become a legitimate source of news and method of communication with a vast international audience. To illustrate, following the Cork air crash in Ireland in 2011, within 1 minute of the crash the news was on Facebook. In health protection we must be aware that news and messages spread fast. If they are not monitored and responded to in a timely manner, then there can be a negative impact upon incident management. It also bypasses traditional media gatekeepers such as newspaper editors, allowing the user to have a direct relationship with the receiver. Journalists now expect public sector organisations to have a social media presence.

From the point of view of health protection, social media is an invaluable resource. Emergency services including the police and ambulance service have used it to great effect to send and receive messages about incidents, using it to:

- Inform
- Respond
- Engage

For example, during civil disturbances in England in 2012, social media was used by the emergency services to inform the public of what was happening and what to do, and also enabled communities to mobilise such as during the clean-up operation. Conversely of course, social media was blamed for mobilising the disturbances in the first place.

Considerations for using social media

While many of the principles governing social media are similar to those required for traditional media, it is important to be aware of a number of unique challenges that using it presents:

- The breadth of people who might read what you say and what is being said about your organisation or an incident is huge. While this may be of benefit in getting your message out, it can be an issue when things go wrong.
- Once posted the message is out there and, for example, in respect of Twitter, even if you are able to delete a post, it doesn't guarantee someone hasn't already seen it or retweeted it (forwarded it to their followers).
- Concern that legal issues might be raised; following an incident you might be asked: 'Why didn't you use social media to communicate or listen to the public/other organisations?' Always be aware of your organisation's media policies and the potential legal implications of what you post.
- Communicating important messages in a few words. Twitter only allows 140 characters per tweet which includes pictures and web links. Formulating effective messages that say what we want them to say, in a way that we want them to be received, is a new and challenging skill.
- Social media allows us to listen as well as inform, react and respond. Using tools like hashtags (#) on Twitter can allow us to monitor public feeling and knowledge about an issue.
- Social media accounts need to be regularly used and maintained to remain useful.
- Social media accounts can blur the divide between personal and professional – it is vital you understand the difference.

- It is important to continue to monitor your posts, as the public may comment and further issues or misinformation may arise from public posts.

Practising public health tip 1.14 Using social media: Consider opportunities to utilise social media in your day-to-day work to help communicate with the public and with stakeholders.

Practising public health tip 1.15 Ending conversations: Toward the end of conversations consider:

- Asking if there are any questions the person would like to ask or any points they would wish to be clarified
- Outlining what happens next, for example, detailing the next steps of an outbreak investigation
- Detailing where and when further information will be available, for example, on local radio for a chemical incident

FURTHER READING

Hawker J et al. 2012. *Communicable Disease Control and Health Protection Handbook*, 3rd ed. Wiley-Blackwell, Oxford, UK.

Health Protection Agency. 2008. *Health Emergency Planning: A Handbook for Practitioners*, 2nd ed.

Heath D, Heath C. 2008. *Made to Stick: Why Some Ideas Take Hold and Others Come Unstuck*. Mashable.com – Social media and technology news.

Mendelson BJ. 2012. *Social Media is Bull****.* St. Martin's Press, New York, NY.

NHS employers: HR and social media. www.nhsemployers.org.

Social media highway code: A guide for GPs. RCGP. www.rcgp.org.uk.

The news: Read, listen and watch a wide variety of news media to understand how the same story can be communicated differently, e.g. *The Guardian* (a broadsheet newspaper) vs. *The Daily Mail* (a tabloid newspaper) vs. the BBC (TV news) in the UK.

Your organisation's media and social media policies.

2

Health promotion

VAL MESSENGER, ANGELA BAKER AND ADAM D M BRIGGS

Introduction 21
Planning a health promotion initiative 22
Effecting individual behaviour change 23
Deciding what to do 23
Putting it into practice 25
Worked through health promotion scenario 33
Further reading 43

PRE-READING

- For an introduction into the theory underlying health promotion, more information can be found in Section 2 of Lewis G, Sheringham J, Lopez Bernal J, and Crayford T, *Mastering Public Health: A Postgraduate Guide to Examinations and Revalidation*, 2nd ed., CRC Press, Boca Raton, Florida, 2014.
- NICE (National Institute for Health and Care Excellence) Public Health Guidance for a range of evidence based interventions for promoting and improving health, categorised both by disease and by risk factor. http://www.nice.org.uk, follow links to guidance, and then public health guidance.
- UK Local Government Association page on health, wellbeing, and adult social care. This has up-to-date information about the organisation of public health and social care in the UK (http://www.local.gov.uk/health-wellbeing-and-adult-social-care).
- Public Health England (PHE) site for latest strategies, frameworks, and resources on health and wellbeing (https://www.gov.uk/government/organisations/public-health-england).
- For more detailed underlying theory of health promotion, the following is an excellent resource: Naidoo J and Wills J, Foundations for Health Promotion, 3rd ed., Elsevier Health Sciences, 2009.

INTRODUCTION

This chapter will explore how health promotion can be integrated into everything public health professionals do, thereby maximising an initiative's health benefit. It provides a refresher of some of the most commonly used health promotion models and frameworks, and how they can be used in practice. Communication is a key aspect of health promotion, as it is the way in which we aim to inform and ultimately affect behaviour change. Such change can be at the individual, group or societal level, and the approach taken and intervention chosen needs to reflect both who we are targeting and what outcome we are trying to achieve.

Before defining what health promotion is, it is important to define health. In 1948, the World

Health Organisation (WHO) constitution defined health as:

> a state of complete physical, social and mental well-being, and not merely the absence of disease or infirmity.

Within the context of health promotion, however, health is considered less as an abstract state (as with the WHO definition) and more as a means to an end, a resource that permits people to lead individually, socially and economically productive lives. The Ottawa Charter for Health Promotion (WHO, 1986) defines *health promotion* as:

> the process of enabling people to increase control over, and to improve their health.

This is a concept that emphasises an individual's social and personal resources as well as physical capabilities to improve health.

This chapter will take you through planning a health promotion initiative, making the right decisions and putting it into practice, before illustrating these concepts with an example.

PLANNING A HEALTH PROMOTION INITIATIVE

When first planning a health promotion initiative, it is crucial to recognise that populations contain different people with different backgrounds and opportunities. These factors will influence both the individual's own health and their response to any health promotion intervention. The work of Dahlgren and Whitehead (1991) demonstrates the multiple factors that influence health (Figure 2.1).

Considering each of these factors in turn helps to identify areas to target health promotion interventions:

The person (the central circle and zone 1) – people are born with inherited factors that determine a certain level of health, and disease risk varies by age and gender. So for example, we know

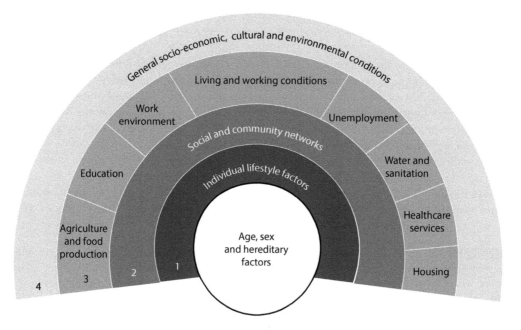

Figure 2.1 Dahlgren and Whitehead's health rainbow. (From Dahlgren G, Whitehead M. (1991). *Policies and Strategies to Promote Social Equity in Health*. Stockholm, Sweden: Institute for Futures Studies. http://www.iffs.se/wp-content/uploads/2011/01/20080109110739filmZ8UVQv2wQFShMRF6cuT.pdf. With permission.)

there are hereditary links to certain cancers such as breast cancer, that males have a higher risk of heart disease than females and that this risk increases with age. Although the underlying risk is given, we can monitor and screen to identify symptoms early and initiate treatment. We can also modify additional risk from unhealthy lifestyles such as increasing levels of physical activity and eating a healthier diet. Knowing that a particular population has an older age demographic, for example, will help guide what type of intervention may be more relevant.

People live in families (zones 1 and 2) – families come in different shapes and sizes and have different beliefs and attitudes to health. The individual living in, or having grown up in, a given family environment may be exposed to passive smoke or be more likely to eat a certain diet which would differ if living elsewhere. These not only impact on the individual's health, but they also impact on the next generation's health. The definition of family will vary for different population groups and cultures.

Families live within communities (zone 2) – communities also impact on health. Important factors to consider include the resources available to those communities, such as is there a park? How close is the road? Is there much crime? Other community influences on health include the value a community places on health, and whether social norms or peer pressure influence certain behaviours like riding a bike to work or buying certain foods, and the support that a community can provide.

Communities are supported by society (zone 3) – the society's structure will impact on health. Is there a readily available supply of food, and what type of food? Is there clean water and is it easy to build exercise into the average day? Does society promote health or does it make being healthy the more difficult choice? How does that society care for older people?

Societal ethos and the political landscape (zone 4) – these also affect health. For example, does the state support healthy choices through legislation or does it instead prefer individualism? This also links to planning – are there green spaces for people to exercise? Are homes well insulated?

EFFECTING INDIVIDUAL BEHAVIOUR CHANGE

There is UK guidance produced by the National Institute for Health and Care Excellence (NICE) that explores how to create a behavioural change strategy (Public Health Guidance 49 at http://www.nice.org.uk). Why people change is covered under Section 'Developing Personal Skills'; however, it is important to understand and build behaviour change strategies into all policies so that every intervention becomes a behaviour change opportunity. Behaviour change through brief interventions should be a core part of all social and healthcare workers, regardless of their role (see Box 2.1).

DECIDING WHAT TO DO

When considering the design of any health promotion initiative, frameworks can help to clarify the mechanism through which an intervention may be having an effect. Choice and enabling healthy decision making is an important principle of health promotion. However, should people have free choice if the impact is to cause poor health that the state has to pay for, or if their behaviour harms others? The intervention ladder published by the Nuffield Council on Bioethics (2007) provides a framework with which to classify different health promotion interventions. Health promotion initiatives can cover all steps of the ladder, even within the same intended health outcome, for example, with efforts to tackle childhood obesity in the UK (Figure 2.2).

EXERCISE 2.1

Using the prevention of skin cancer, rather than the childhood obesity example presented in Figure 2.2, try to think of eight levels of intervention on the Nuffield Council on Bioethics intervention ladder (*hint*: consider sunbed legislation).

Alongside the Nuffield Council on Bioethics intervention ladder, the Beattie typology model of health promotion (Beattie, 1991) provides a

BOX 2.1: Brief interventions and making every contact count

Brief interventions are interventions that take a short amount of time and are often done in addition to the primary reason for a given patient/professional interaction, for example, a dentist asking about smoking during a routine appointment and giving details of how to get help to quit. Brief interventions can take different forms and are generally used to provide information and advice about an unhealthy behaviour, and to provide options for how to access further help and support.

An example in the UK is Making Every Contact Count (MECC; http://www.makingeverycontactcount.co.uk/). The premise of MECC, like other programmes focused on brief interventions, is that every contact someone has with a member of the public is an opportunity to improve health. You do not have to be a health professional to be able to act; you simply need to know what questions to ask, what basic advice to give and where to signpost people for more information and help. Brief interventions are developing an increasingly strong evidence base on how they can improve population health, and MECC is now recommended by the UK Department of Health as something that all UK health professionals should be practising.

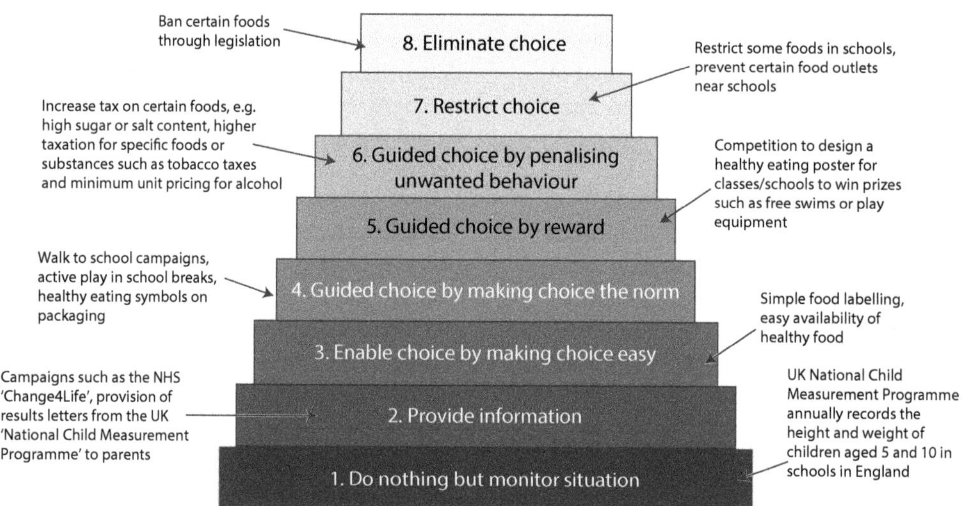

Figure 2.2 Nuffield Council on Bioethics intervention ladder with examples of interventions to tackle childhood obesity. (Nuffield Council on Bioethics. 2007. *Public Health: Ethical Issues*. London: Nuffield Council on Bioethics. http://nuffieldbioethics.org/wp-content/uploads/2014/07/Public-health-ethical-issues.pdf. With permission.)

framework to explore the context of a health promotion strategy in terms of individual versus collective (the focus of the intervention) and authoritarian versus negotiated (the mode of intervention) approaches (Figure 2.3).

To maximise population behaviour change for a particular risk factor, the strategies implemented should aim to affect all four quadrants of the Beattie model. For example, Figure 2.4 illustrates an intervention aimed at reducing smoking.

EXERCISE 2.2

The use of frameworks and models can help ensure that you consider the full range of interventions available to you. Choose a health promotion intervention you are familiar with and map interventions to the four quadrants of the Beattie model (as has been done for smoking in Figure 2.4).

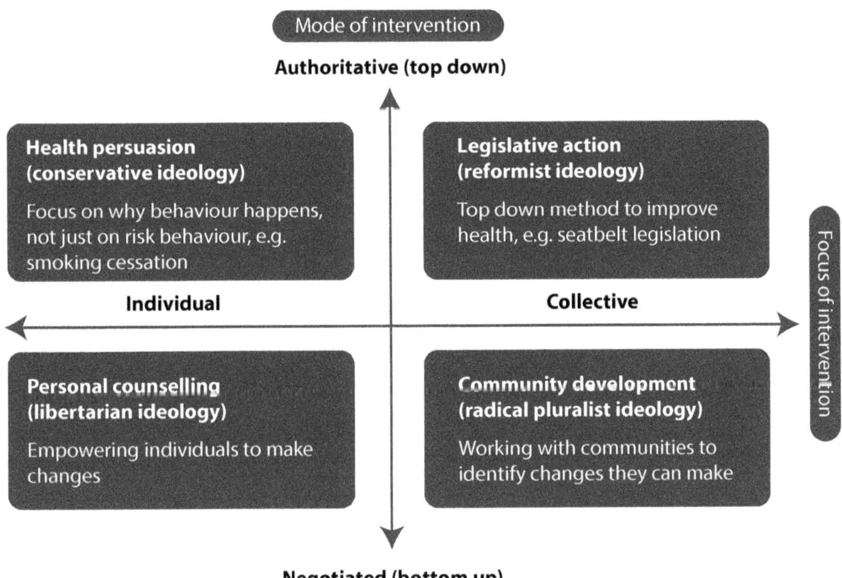

Figure 2.3 Beattie's typology model of health promotion. (From Beattie, A., *The Sociology of the Health Service*, Routledge, London, 1991. With permission.)

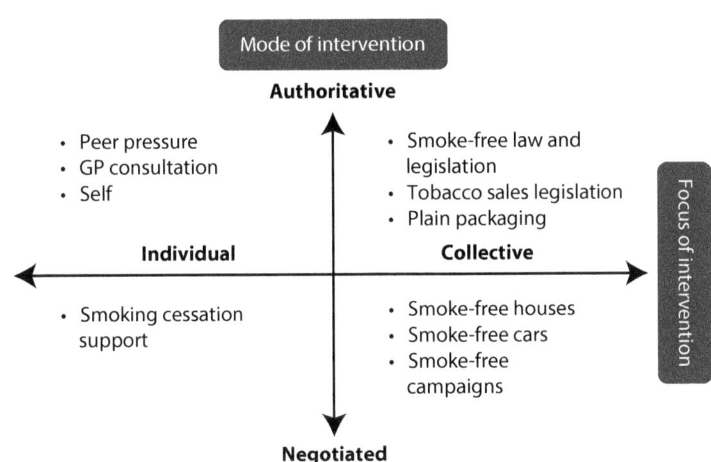

Figure 2.4 Interventions to reduce smoking, categorised in Beattie's model of health promotion.

Box 2.2 discusses how nudge theory can be used to improve health.

PUTTING IT INTO PRACTICE

Using the Ottawa Charter for Health Promotion (WHO, 1986), we will examine health promotion as a topic through five types of intervention:

- Building healthy public policy
- Creating a supportive environment
- Strengthening community action
- Developing personal skills
- Re-orientating health services

To create an effective health promotion strategy or plan, it is important to think about and develop all five themes.

BOX 2.2: Nudge

Thaler and Sunstein's 2008 book *Nudge: Improving Decisions about Health, Wealth, and Happiness* has created a considerable stir among decision makers looking to improve health without 'nannying' the public. The book highlights the potential benefits of making interventions aimed at steps 2–4 of the Nuffield Council on Bioethics intervention ladder (Figure 2.2). Examples of nudges include traffic light labels on food packaging giving the consumer instantly recognisable colour-coded advice on the quantities of unhealthy nutrients in the product, changing the default dessert in a canteen to fruit instead of custard, or putting up signs saying how 98% of visitors to a hospital choose not to smoke.

When thinking about public health interventions, nudge theory provides a useful way of expanding the range of ways you can improve people's behaviour, alongside other interventions in the Nuffield Council on Bioethics ladder.

Buliding healthy public policy

The *Oxford English Dictionary's* definition of *policy* is

> *A principle or course of action adopted or proposed as desirable, advantageous, or expedient.*

Healthy public policy improves equity and population health alongside delivering the policy's primary aim. For example:

- A transport policy sets out how transport will be delivered to people.
- A healthy public transport policy sets out how transport will be delivered considering both the health impacts of transportation and equality issues. Such a strategy may consider environmental issues and green transport options as potentially impacting on health, as well as equality of access such as disabled access and provision of services in deprived areas.

Policies that are explicitly designed for health may also need to work across multiple sectors. For example, a healthy eating policy for a deprived community will require cooperation from a range of sectors. These could include city planning regarding the licensing of fast food vans and the education department in order to influence the provision of school food.

All those involved in policy making should consider the impact of the policy on health and health inequalities; furthermore, the policy should be evaluated regarding its impact on health. Box 2.3 outlines the steps required and Figure 2.5 summarises the cycle of developing healthy public policy.

ACTION FOR PUBLIC HEALTH TEAMS

Influencing a policy has the potential to significantly improve the health of a population with minimal expenditure. Public health teams should know how to influence policy within their local area, and not just policies that are seen as part of the public health portfolio. In an organisation with a large number of policies, it may be necessary to prioritise a limited public health resource and aim to influence those policies with the greatest potential health impact.

Health impact assessments (HIAs) are an effective way of assessing a policy for health benefits; Figure 2.6 outlines the HIA procedure. HIAs help to ensure that any potentially negative health impacts are mitigated against and positive health impacts are maximised. HIAs can greatly improve communication with the public as the process can assist stakeholders (including the public) to input into the development of policy. There are various resources and examples that can help you design your own HIA tool, many of which can be found through the WHO website (WHO, 2014): http://www.who.int/hia/en/.

Finally, when designing a policy, it is important to set realistic and measurable outcomes – a policy is unlikely to change or improve health if there is no way of measuring its success. Therefore you should develop an evaluation plan while the policy is being drafted; this needs to identify what success will look like and have clear ways to measure it.

BOX 2.3: Developing healthy public policy

Vision – what do you want to achieve from your policy? Senior support will be key to ensuring that your vision can be delivered.

Beliefs and values – what do you believe and value about the policy; why bother? Framing the message of the policy to stakeholders is important so that the health benefits can be reinforced and counter any negatives such as reduced choice.

Support for your policy – is your policy important to other people and do you have organisational buy-in? Engaging the target population will ensure the success of the policy, allowing you to get feedback and make it culturally appropriate.

Draft your policy – outline the background to your policy; what are the main drivers for the policy? Clarify the desired outcomes and the proposed interventions to get you there, as well as how the policy will be implemented, monitored and evaluated.

Consult on your policy – develop your policy to be acceptable and achievable. This means engaging not just with your target population but also with other groups and organisations affected such as primary care teams or local community groups.

Organisational sign-off for the policy – so it becomes the expected behaviour.

Implementation plan – including training and education. This may also benefit from working with your internal communications team to draft a press release and speak to local radio.

Monitor – is the policy being followed and how are you 'policing' the policy?

Evaluate and reassess policy – modify the policy to make it more effective.

Source: Adapted from Public Health Ontario. 2013. The eight steps to developing healthy public policy. Ontario.

Creating a supportive environment

Some neighbourhoods have good access to fresh and affordable food; others have only fast food outlets, off licenses, and convenience stores. How people live and what is available to them within their environment has an overarching impact on their health. Providing people with healthy choices means providing a supportive environment.

> The choices we make are shaped by the choices we have (Rogow et al., 2008)

Supportive environments are relevant to health promotion in specific settings; these may be schools, hospitals, workplaces and cities. A supportive environment is one that:

- Offers people protection from the factors that can threaten good health
- Fosters participation in health and enables people to expand their capabilities and health self-reliance
- Makes the healthy choice the easy choice
- Is critical for a person-centred approach to health and the healthcare services which are available to them

Actions to create supportive environments for promoting health have many facets and can cover all aspects of both the Beattie model (Figure 2.3) and the Nuffield Council on Bioethics ladder of intervention (Figure 2.2). Examples include:

- Tobacco control legislation, plain packaging and smoke-free places
- Changes in alcohol legislation and single-unit minimum pricing
- Banning unhealthy food outlets close to schools
- Ensuring access to exercise facilities for all by supporting women from certain ethnic backgrounds to exercise in female-only settings
- Implementing stress management programs in the workplace for staff
- Promoting community participation through provision of communal space and facilities

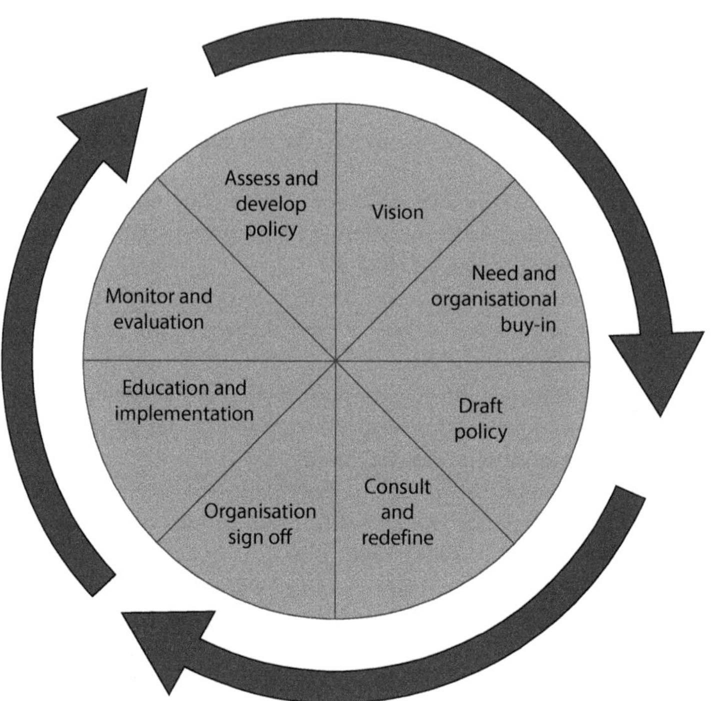

Figure 2.5 The cycle for developing healthy public policy. (Adapted from Public Health Ontario. 2013. The eight steps to developing healthy public policy. Ontario.)

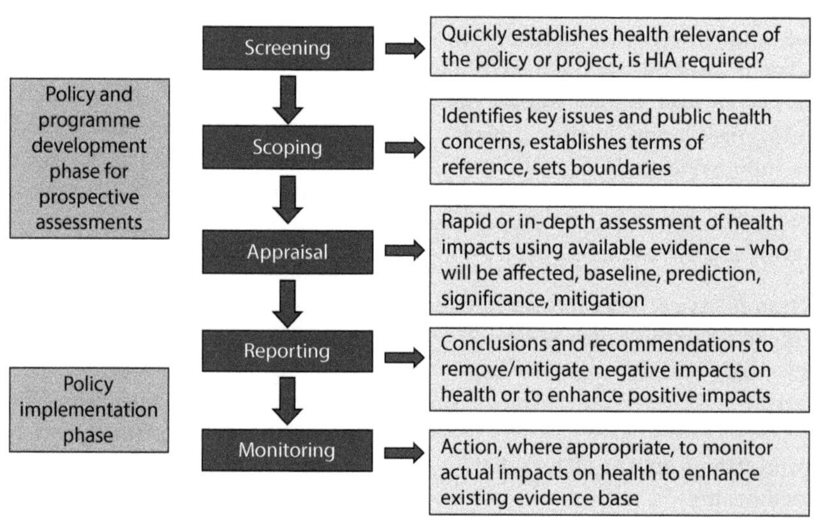

Figure 2.6 Health impact assessment procedure. (Adapted from World Health Organisation. 2014. The HIA procedure. Geneva: WHO. http://www.who.int/hia/tools/process/en.)

- Strengthening the links between health and environmental strategies by introducing cycle tracks and maintaining pavements to encourage active travel
- Introducing community-based interventions for a range of lifestyle issues, e.g. health checks, smoking cessation programmes and slimming programmes
- Making health services welcoming and accessible, with friendly staff, seating, play areas for children and access to drinking water
- Improving equitable access to health through initiatives such as promoting sexual health and wellbeing for people with disabilities

ACTION FOR PUBLIC HEALTH TEAMS

Public health professionals are well placed to develop supportive environments by:

- Influencing their own workplace by promoting staff health, including ensuring that personnel and service contracts place the expectation for staff health on employers
- Championing the use of contracts to ensure public services are delivered in smoke-free sites
- Directly or indirectly commissioning programmes which are accessible and address lifestyle issues as well as health-related issues

Strengthening community action

The *Oxford English Dictionary's* definition of *community* is

> A body of people who live in the same place, usually sharing a common cultural or ethnic identity.

People can belong to multiple communities: the street they live on, a specific ethnicity or culture within which they resonate, a particular faith group or gender group.

In the UK, the Localism Act 2011 and the Equality Act 2010 both aim to break down barriers within communities and neighbourhoods by encouraging local decisions to be made to suit local need (such as social housing development or local planning decisions) and outlawing discrimination against individuals on the basis of gender, ethnicity, age, sexual orientation, religion or disability. Legislation alone will not make communities stronger, and instead it is a tool to support community action.

A supportive community is a community that members feel they belong to and that they personally have an interest in being a part of; it will prosper and thrive as people work together to achieve a common aim. A supportive community can readily facilitate the work of public health teams through:

1. Addressing a community's concerns to improve health
2. Delivering public health messages
3. Understanding risks to health and how to mitigate them

Communities are fluid and contain multiple assets, including people, green spaces, community buildings and environmental and financial resources. The public health goal when working with communities and supporting their development is for any community health-promoting action to be self-sustaining as far as possible. This enables the longevity of the intervention and gives the community ownership of, and a stake in, the initiative.

ACTION FOR PUBLIC HEALTH TEAMS

When working with different communities, public health professionals should support the growth of community spirit. This can be achieved through:

- Supporting and developing community volunteers and champions
- Using specific tools available to public health, such as local government or community committees (an example would be the Health and Wellbeing Board in England) to support local health policy and community development
- Using and influencing existing community action to get the most out of outcomes
- Encouraging communities to become self-supporting and more resilient

Developing personal skills

Health promotion can allow individuals to develop their own skills to make healthy choices and positive lifestyle changes. Lifestyle change is defined as *any modification or transformation which impacts on a person's behaviour* and is influenced by a range of factors.

The stages of change model (Figure 2.7) can help public health professionals to develop effective behaviour change interventions.

The stages of change model has six stages:

1. *Precontemplation* – the person does not recognise the need to change or does not believe that their behaviour has a harmful impact on their health. At this stage, people do not have any intention of changing within the next 6 months.
2. *Contemplation* – the person recognises they have a problem and are considering change. People in this stage may plan to change and begin to think about how change can be brought about but are not ready to commit.
3. *Preparation* – the person has committed to make the change and has a plan for how the change is going to be made.
4. *Action* – the change is instigated.
5. *Maintenance* – the behaviour change has been adopted and the person is trying to maintain the new behaviour. The behaviour is becoming normalised and the lifestyle change becomes embedded.
6. *Relapse* – at any stage the person can relapse and the unwanted behaviour can become dominant again.

When designing a health promotion initiative aimed at individuals, the stages of change model provides a framework to design the scope of the initiative: Will it target individuals to move between two particular stages, or will it work across the entire model?

In order to help guide this decision, it is important to assess the target population's readiness for change – where those being targeted currently exist within the stages of change model. Table 2.1

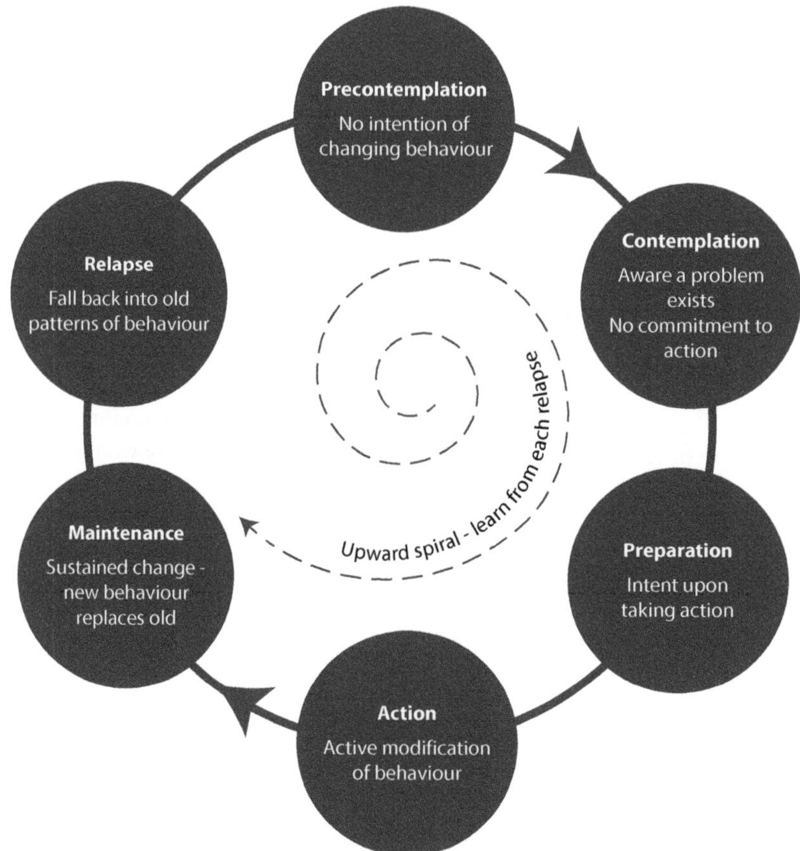

Figure 2.7 The stages of change model. (From Prochaska JO and DiClemente CC. 1984. *Advances in Cancer Control – 1983*. New York: Alan R. Liss. With permission.)

Table 2.1 Identifying an individual's readiness to change their behaviour, and possible public health approaches

Behaviour	Action of individual	Stage	Examples of support
Consciousness raising	Becoming aware of an issue through persistent messaging over time and through different mediums	Precontemplation Contemplation	Information, awareness raising especially by people in positions of trust
Self-revalidation	Feeling uncomfortable about weight, smoking and alcohol consumption and a feeling that action is required to reduce risks	Precontemplation Contemplation	Information about the options for treatment/ change support available, information about benefits of change
Self-liberation	Committing to make a change, beginning to work out how the change can be maintained and looking forward to starting	Contemplation Preparation	Support to make plans which will work, help to identify potential high-risk points so difficult situations can be managed
Counter-conditioning	Substituting alternatives for behaviour, drinking water instead of snacking or having sweets instead of smoking	Preparation Action	Support to identify substitutions which support and promote health, so how to avoid snacking while giving up smoking
Stimulus control	Avoid high-risk situations such as going out and meeting with friends that smoke	Action Maintenance	Support to identify triggers which may lead to relapse, techniques for managing flash points
Reinforcing management	Rewarding oneself for achieving a goal, having contracts with self such as buying new clothes when losing weight	Action Maintenance	Support to identify rewards which support and promote health; this may include shopping but not if may cause financial distress
Helpful relationships	Being open and working with people who can support the changed behaviour	All stages	Support to identify people who help and people who don't
Dramatic relief	Playing out one's feelings, becoming an anti-smoker, telling people how many calories are in specific foods	All stages, when there is a chance of relapse	Helping people recognise that this is part of the process of change and who 'helpful' people are that can help manage change
Environmental re-evaluation	Changing lifestyle to accommodate new behaviours, to embed behaviours into new ways of life	All stages	Positive reinforcement about changes and their impact such as health gains and environmental gains; link to people's own values
Social liberation	Self-empowered, being at ease with new behaviours	Maintenance	Recognise and reinforce achievements through positive messaging

identifies the behaviours adopted by individuals at different stages of change alongside examples of the support that can be useful for those individuals, thereby informing the design of a health promotion initiative that specifically develops personal skills.

EXERCISE 2.3

Relating back to Exercise 2.1, consider someone who sunbathes without the use of protective lotion and who regularly uses sunbeds in the winter. How would you support them to change their behaviour through the various steps of the stages of change model?

The health belief model (Hochbaum, 1958) can also be useful when designing a health promotion initiative to develop personal skills. The stages of change model can be used to plan the scope of the initiative, and the health belief model (see Table 2.2) can be used to explore different motivators and barriers to changing a particular behaviour, as well as identify mechanisms to promote healthy behaviour change.

Re-orientating health services

Recently there have been numerous reports that health services across the globe are becoming overwhelmed by ill-health and need to cope with rising patient demands: services may need to change to continue to be sustainable. In England, for example, the Wanless Report (Wanless, 2004) highlighted the need to move to what was described as a fully engaged scenario to manage the increasing demand of an aging population, a growing population and an expanding number of treatments and medical interventions. Within public health, this fully engaged scenario means:

Table 2.2 Health belief model

Health belief	Explanation	Actions
Perceived susceptibility	An individual's assessment of their risk of getting the condition	Highlight risks among the target population, both of the behaviour being targeted and of related undesirable outcomes of the behaviour
Perceived severity	An individual's assessment of the seriousness of the condition, and its potential consequences	Provide education about the implications of the condition, both to the individual and the wider family, community or society
Perceived barriers	An individual's assessment of the influences that facilitate or discourage adoption of the promoted behaviour	Identify barriers and act to remove them
Perceived benefits	An individual's assessment of the positive consequences of adopting the behaviour	Highlight the expected benefits to the individual and the population of the change in behaviour
Cues to action	Triggers for an individual to make a change	Provide information on how to change behaviours, promote awareness
Self-efficacy	An individual's ability to act and make a change	Offer guidance or training on how to act, and a support structure once the new behaviour is adopted

Source: From Hochbaum GM. 1958. *Public Participation in Medical Screening Programs: A Socio-Psychological Study.* PHS no. 572. Washington, DC: U.S. Government Printing Office. With permission.

- Ensuring the population is healthier and therefore needing less care
- Having suitable and effective self-care alternatives so that people are able to take more responsibility for their own health
- Providing an effective evidence base and developing best practice guidance to disseminate and promote effective health service design

ACTION FOR PUBLIC HEALTH TEAMS

In order to facilitate the re orientating of health services to a focus on prevention, public health professionals can consider the following:

- Using the behaviour change evidence base to commission services that promote health
- Ensuring health promotion initiatives are properly evaluated so that they can add to the evidence base
- Working with and influencing clinical commissioners to develop the early stages of a clinical pathway, thereby ensuring that health improvement services are available (see Box 2.4)

BOX 2.4: The commissioning cycle

The commissioning cycle demonstrates how the frameworks and models described in this chapter can translate into everyday practice. The commissioning cycle, as described by the UK National Audit Office (2014), has five elements:

1. Assessing needs
2. Designing and re-designing services
3. Sourcing providers
4. Delivery
5. Monitoring and evaluation

In order to inform the development of each stage, there is a need for public, customer and provider feedback.

Practising public health tip 2.1 Commissioning services: In some health economies public health teams commission services. The steps in the commissioning cycle are similar except that once the service is designed, the team goes through a procedure of commercial tendering (going out to market) to identify appropriate service providers. This is intended to allow open competition and drive down costs.

EXERCISE 2.4

Consider a proposal for a drug education intervention aimed at young people using the commissioning cycle. Think of two points for each of the five steps outlined in Box 2.4.

WORKED THROUGH HEALTH PROMOTION SCENARIO

In this scenario we will examine the implementation of a health improvement initiative to tackle high rates of teenage pregnancy. It will develop with increasing amounts of information being provided. The examples are designed to be directly applicable to different aspects of public health practice.

Practising public health tip 2.2 Using behaviour change models: You may find it helpful to structure your answers around a behaviour change model that you are confident with. Consider the audience you are told you will be presenting to when you are identifying what information from the situation you think is most relevant to communicate. Also think what additional advice, views or information you will want to elicit from them. As with all scenarios, be sure to use your listening skills and ensure that the person you are speaking with understands the points you are trying to make.

Triggers for initiating a health improvement intervention

Attention can be drawn to a topic that could benefit from a health improvement intervention for a number of reasons. These include:

- An organisation missing a performance target
- Political intervention – question from a national or local politician
- Stakeholder concerns – head teacher, general practitioner (GP), school health nurse
- Another department/organisation raising concerns, e.g. department of education or a local school
- A problem identified through routine surveillance of health indicators
- The launch of a relevant national campaign or policy

Practising public health tip 2.3 Triggers for interventions: The trigger (if described) may help you focus your initial response to a problem and make it specifically relevant to the need for intervention.

In practice, it may not be immediately obvious from a problem, or question, that the solution lies in carrying out a needs assessment or implementing a health promotion intervention; e.g. 'How can we turn around this performance indicator'?

Assimilation and use of information

Assimilation of information is a key aspect of health promotion. Through analysis of data, the need for a health promotion initiative may be identified; furthermore, it will also provide information to help target the relevant population.

In this scenario, a sexual health needs assessment identified that despite teenage conception rates in the region being lower than the national average, they were not reducing at the rate seen in the rest of England or in statistical neighbours. Local rates showed decreases in more affluent localities and increases in more deprived localities. In addition, there were geographical hotspots where conception rates were consistently in the highest 20% of wards in England. A small number of secondary schools had catchment populations that covered these hotspots.

Practising public health tip 2.4 Benchmarking performance: Statistical neighbours are comparator organisations that are deemed suitable for benchmarking against because of similarities to your organisation. They may also be referred to as peer groups. When benchmarking your local area's performance, they can be a useful tool to discuss and be aware of.

Additional facts identified in the needs assessment include:

- Nearly half of teenage conceptions in the region end in abortion (more in the under 16s).
- 12% of abortions to women aged 18 years and under are second abortions.
- There is an association between teenage pregnancy and educational attainment.
- Only around 1 in 5 teenage mothers continue in education, employment or training.

Practising public health tip 2.5 Different data sources: In a scenario like this, the information presented has come from secondary analyses of data; it is important for you to acknowledge this when discussing with colleagues or stakeholders. Also, when discussing an intervention with colleagues, you should highlight the importance of considering the views of the target population. In addition, extra knowledge may be available through a literature review or best practice examples.

Consulting young people

Consulting the target population of any health promotion intervention can be an extremely valuable source of information. For example, information in this scenario that came from consulting young people includes the following findings:

- One-third of young people in school reported that they have had sexual intercourse.
- The average age for first reported intercourse was 14½ years.
- Two-thirds of young people felt under pressure to have sex.
- Of those who were sexually active, only 16% had planned to have intercourse before it happened the first time.

Young people wanted sex education that included:

- Time to discuss scenarios and how to cope with emotions
- Relationship skills, e.g. making informed choices, decision making, negotiation, saying yes or no
- Accurate information about contraception including information about services and where to access them
- Young people's rights to confidentiality
- Acknowledgement that boys need to know about contraception as well as girls
- Improved provision of information, advice and support in school

Desired services included those that:

- Offer young-people-only sessions
- Allow the person to see the same professional each time they visit
- Act as a drop-in for a lot of different health issues
- Give the opportunity to help decide how a clinic should run
- Provide group sessions on sexual health and relationships
- Offer more accessible services including increased availability on the weekends

EXERCISE 2.5

Think of a health promotion intervention to reduce teenage pregnancy rates using the information above. How do the points listed impact on the design of your intervention?

Using the literature

In this example, a research question and a search strategy were developed to identify the long-term social and health outcomes for a teenage mother and their child. A key skill in public health is being able to ask a research question, develop a search strategy and document search terms. Such a search will often provide useful information for identifying a target outcome for a health promotion intervention, as well as inform any future related work.

In this scenario, the literature review found that teenage mothers were

- Less likely to complete education
- More likely to live in poverty
- More likely to be unsupported by the child's father
- More likely to smoke while pregnant
- More likely to live in poor housing
- More likely to experience post-natal depression

The search also found that their children were:

- More likely to be born premature
- More likely have low birth weight
- More likely to be exposed to tobacco smoke
- At increased risk of emotional and behavioural disorders
- At increased risk of abuse or neglect
- More likely to have low educational attainment
- More likely to live in social deprivation
- More likely to have little or no contact with father
- More likely to become a teenage parent

EXERCISE 2.6

How could this information affect either the design or the delivery of the health promotion intervention you designed in Exercise 2.5 (consider where you may implement an intervention and what would be your target population)?

After you have done this, see the main text and practising public health tips below for how the scenario may unfold.

Learning from elsewhere

The UK Department of Education and Skills (2006) identified risk factors for teenage pregnancy, as shown diagrammatically in Table 2.3.

EXERCISE 2.7

How does Table 2.3 add to or reinforce what you did in Exercise 2.6?

Understanding your audience

In presenting a health promotion proposal, it is important to consider how to engage relevant stakeholders and identify what their motivations may be. As a public health professional, you may be required to influence the immediate audience or present a proposal aimed at a different audience. For the teenage pregnancy scenario some examples of stakeholders and their motivations are provided in Table 2.4.

Table 2.3 Risk factors for teenage pregnancy identified by the UK Department for Education and Skills (2006)

	Deprivation	
Risk-taking behaviour	**Education**	**Social circumstances**
Poor and inconsistent use of contraception	Low educational attainment	Daughter of a teenage mother
Alcohol and substance misuse	Dislike of/not attending school	Living in care
Previous pregnancy or abortion	Leaving school at 16 with no qualifications	Ethnicity
Poor mental health		Parental aspirations
Involvement in crime		
Early onset of sexual activity		

Table 2.4 Possible motivations of different stakeholders to support a health promotion initiative aimed at reducing teenage pregnancy rates

Stakeholder	Possible motivations
Chief executive officer (CEO) – local government authority	Achieving performance targets; improved educational attainment; more young people in employment, education or training; cost savings with regard to supporting young teenage mothers; positive press
CEO – health commissioner	Achieving a performance target; saving money due to less terminations and births; positive press (particularly if successful)
Head teachers	Reduced school absence; improved educational attainment; support to young people in their care
Teacher	Increased knowledge and access to professional support to advise young people in their care
Health professional, e.g. school health nurse	Ability to deliver a needed service in a supportive environment
Young people	Access to the services and support they had identified through consultation; e.g. they said 'we would like more services in schools' and we said 'we will ensure that a school health nurse is in school every day'

Handling uncertainty and conflict

In practice there are often uncertainties and conflicts related to implementing a health promotion proposal. Consultation with both potential users of the service and key stakeholders can help identify conflict at an early stage. When identified, issues and risks can be documented and mitigating actions can be taken. However, always be prepared for an unexpected issue to arise.

An example of a health promotion initiative may be to have a named school health nurse in schools located in areas of high teenage pregnancy rates who is able to provide contraception advice and support. Alongside this, a text messaging service may be made available all year round which is answered by a school health nurse within 24 hours. An alternative intervention could be the ability for teachers to signpost students to a school health nurse or contraception service in a local community setting.

In this example, uncertainties and areas of conflict, along with potential mitigating actions when communicating with stakeholders, are shown in Table 2.5.

Given the potential uncertainties outlined above, it is important to describe what success would look like and what an alternative intervention may be. In this example, success may be defined as 80% of schools taking up the initiative with at least half of the schools doing so within the first year.

Packaging the message

The message may need to be packaged, or framed, and shared differently with different stakeholders. The underlying information and message should be consistent, but different facts may be used depending on who the message is aimed at.

Table 2.5 Potential areas of conflict that could be encountered along with some mitigating actions

Uncertainty/area of conflict	Potential mitigating strategy
The preferred location for delivering any intervention was identified as within local schools, but head teachers' views on this were unknown.	Head teachers may respond well to an approach from the CEOs of local health organisations and local government. You could suggest that you will provide a letter to include a brief outline of the issue and an offer of a meeting with the local health organisations where information will be presented and where there would be opportunities for discussion.
Initial discussions with local stakeholders, such as teachers, councillors or the general public, showed that when they thought of teenage conceptions they immediately thought of teenage mums, i.e. those young women who chose to continue with their pregnancy.	Clarify what is meant by conceptions and what proportion end in terminations.
The data suggests that it may be better to have a targeted intervention, to be only put in place in selected schools in high-risk areas. This could be challenged by the press, other head teachers and local government councillors.	Communicate the data in lay terms to highlight the areas of greatest need. Be open about the fact that resources are limited and that the decisions have been made on the basis of need.
Some members of faith schools may be inhibited with some aspects of the proposal due to religious beliefs and be under pressure externally, e.g. from parent groups and community faith leaders.	Offer a tailored approach in discussion with head teachers.

Practising public health tip 2.6 Clear proposals: Make sure that any proposal is clear. What will be provided, at what cost (if known), where and when?

For example, the health promotion initiative may be to provide additional support in selected schools from school health nurses. Key information will include the nurses being additionally trained in contraception and a text message service being available during school holidays. Additionally, support will be offered to schools to improve the quality of personal health and social education (PHSE) for both boys and girls. This will incur no cost to schools, but they will be expected to revise their PHSE lessons and encourage signposting to the school health nurses. The target time frame is for the intervention to be in place by the autumn term.

Identifying key messages can be helpful when talking to other stakeholders who may need to be convinced about the need for the health promotion initiative. As far as possible, try to tailor advice to the stakeholder's own priorities. For example, with health commissioners it may be helpful to highlight the savings in terms of reduced costs on termination and maternity services, and with the local government you could highlight the potential for improved educational attainment, numbers of people in education, employment or training, and reduced social care costs in supporting young mums.

EXERCISE 2.8

How would you summarise the data provided earlier in this scenario and the rationale for action? Think of the three key messages you would want to highlight to the following stakeholders: a health commissioner; a member of local government; and the press.

Practising public health tip 2.7 Using three key messages: If speaking to the media about the need for a health promotion intervention, you should try and identify three key messages that can summarise the problem, the initiative and the potential impact. For this scenario, three key messages might be

1. Teenage conceptions in the area are not decreasing in line with the rest of England and statistical neighbours.
2. There are particular hotspots where, if action was targeted, not only would conceptions decrease but also there would be other positive benefits such as an improvement in young people's life chances, educational attainment and employment.
3. This is as an important local opportunity to improve the life chances of young people.

Listening and reacting

Listening is a key public health skill. Effective listening can reduce misunderstandings and stress, and lead to improved outcomes (see "Practising public health tip 2.8" on non-verbal communication). Table 2.6 identifies possible conversation scenarios and challenges when discussing a proposed health promotion intervention to reduce teenage pregnancy rates. Effective listening can help identify unwanted situations early and avoid unnecessary conflict.

Potential implementation problems

SOURCING PROVIDERS

It is important to consider how an intervention will be commissioned. National reforms in the

Practising public health tip 2.8 Non-verbal communication: Successful communication – listening, non-verbal communication, managing stress and emotional awareness.

1. *Listening skills:* Listening is one of the most important aspects of effective communication.
   By successful listening, we mean

   a. Understanding the words.
   b. Understanding the information.
   c. Understanding how the speaker feels about what they're communicating.

   Effective listening means that the person speaking feels

   a. That they have been heard and understood.
   b. Safe in communicating their viewpoint, even if it is at odds with the listener.

   Effective listening will

   a. Save time as there are likely to be less misunderstandings and conflicts are addressed early.
   b. Reduce stress as it can help to calm down the speaker, making them feel their concerns have been heard.
   c. Lead to improved outcomes and solutions which meet more people's needs.

   To listen effectively

   a. Ensure that you are focused on the speaker, that they have time and space to get their message over.
   b. Be interested, ask relevant questions.
   c. Do not interrupt, but do ask questions at the end to ensure clarity.
   d. Do not be judgemental.
   e. Do not tell personal stories.

2. *Non-verbal communication:* Our body language tells the speaker a lot about what we are doing and thinking, and whether we are interested in their concerns. Keeping an open stance, using eye contact and sitting forward can help you get more out of the conversation, and help the speaker share their real issues.
   To better read non-verbal communication

   a. Observe people.
   b. Be aware of cultural differences.
   c. Look for a range of signals from a person, rather than reading lots into a single gesture.

   In order to improve your non-verbal communication

   a. Ensure your gestures match up, so that the person feels you are genuine; for example, don't say something that is really sad while smiling.
   b. Use body language to convey positive feedback.

3. *Managing stress:* Stress, when overwhelming, can hamper communication by preventing clarity of thought, your ability to think creatively to solve problems and your ability to act rationally.

To deal with stress during communication

a. Try to recognise when you are becoming stressed.
b. Take a moment to calm down by breathing deeply, and acknowledge that you are feeling uncomfortable.
c. Look for humour in the situation, but be careful not to alienate the other person or persons by making them feel humiliated or that they are not being taken seriously.
d. Look for common ground and work on how to take that forward.
e. Agree to disagree; if necessary,
    i. Take time away from the situation so everyone can calm down by taking a break.
    ii. Physically moving away or finding a quiet place to regain your balance can quickly reduce stress.

4. *Emotional awareness:* Emotional awareness and the ability to manage all of your feelings appropriately is the basis for effective communication.
   Emotional awareness helps you

a. Understand who you are communicating with and their motivation to act
b. Understand yourself and what your personal preferences and barriers might be
c. Understand what is driving you both and where the common grounds might be
d. Communicate clearly and effectively, even when delivering negative messages
e. Build strong, trusting and rewarding relationships, think creatively, solve problems and resolve conflicts

Claude Steiner (1997) breaks emotional literacy into five parts:

1. Knowing your feelings
2. Having a sense of empathy
3. Learning to manage our emotions
4. Repairing emotional damage
5. Putting it all together: emotional interactivity

health service can mean changes to commissioning responsibilities, and different organisations within the health service may have different commissioning rules. This should be considered and factored into any plans for implementation. It is also important to consider opportunities for having the initiative provided by the voluntary and community sector.

KEEPING ON MESSAGE

Health promotion initiatives can often be supported through large-scale social media campaigns. When setting up something local, it is important to consider what is being planned nationally to assess if the same message, branding and themes can be used to provide an opportunity to have local messages reinforced by national media.

Teenage pregnancy and the provision of contraception to young people, particularly to those under 16 years, can be politically very sensitive, and sometimes the press can sensationalise this, particularly the issue of informed consent versus parental knowledge.

Evaluation and monitoring

A common problem with health promotion is a lack of evidence base for interventions as there are few published health promotion randomised controlled trials. Although it is worth noting that as

Table 2.6 Potential scenarios that may arise with different stakeholders when discussing a health promotion initiative to reduce teenage pregnancy rates

Stakeholder	Possible situations	Key considerations	What success would look like
Young person	'It won't happen to me' 'I can't change now, I am too busy and stressed' 'Everyone does it' 'I've tried before and failed'	Presenting local data to make it 'feel real' Maintaining confidentiality but being honest about safeguarding responsibilities Understanding different contraception options and who to ask Developing the stakeholder's skills in relationships and negotiation is as important as giving them facts about sex and contraception Appreciating that any intervention in this area is not just about girls	The stakeholder understanding the risks of unprotected sex Improved confidence in young people to make the right decisions for themselves and to respect other people's decisions Improved uptake of contraception services Increased consultations with teachers or health professionals
Media	Sensationalising contraception provision with or without parental consent Stigmatising young women who get pregnant	Provide facts along with evidence of best practice Provide data, or examples, of de-stigmatisation	Positive press commentary on the new service Public health messages highlighted in media
Other health professionals	'I have no time to deliver health promotion initiatives' 'Who is going to pay for the extra work?'	Health promotion can mean prevention and can be brief Health promotion is aligned with and complements other work streams such as provision of sexual health services and chlamydia screening; it just has a different emphasis	Supported delivery of the health promotion initiative by people working with young people as part of the day job
Local politician	Unpopular or politically sensitive topic Savings in the 'wrong' place, not a priority Need for quick fixes and outcomes Driven by electorate demand rather than population need	Message doesn't need to be labelled as 'sex education' Benefits will be seen across the system (education and employment) and not just within sexual health Awareness is immediate even if outcomes can only be demonstrated in the longer term Support and resources for young people are popular	Politician clear about the positive message for the electorate and happy to be a spokesperson

Practising public health tip 2.9 Using the media: When communicating your message it is important to consider what the aim of the communication is and develop an appropriate communication strategy. Is it to make people aware of a particular issue, to provide information, to provide advice or to change behaviour? If we take an example of high incidence of skin cancer identified in the local population, the use of media could be very different if you want to inform adults what to do if they have a suspicious mole versus encouraging young people to take sun safety precautions.

Social marketing is an additional approach to consider. This approach uses concepts from commercial marketing and the social sciences to develop activities aimed at changing or maintaining people's behaviour to benefit individuals and populations. Social marketing aims to change or maintain how people behave – not what they think or how aware they are of an issue.

Each type of media has its own strengths and weaknesses, and the most common mistake is not to systematically consider which media to use and why. For example, what is the profile of the listeners of your local radio stations or the readership of your local newspapers? A campaign about keeping warm in winter would be best aired on a radio station listened to by an older adult population rather than a music channel preferred by teenagers. Using the local press may seem appropriate, but you must consider which populations are likely to buy and read the paper.

More detail on working with the media can be found in Chapter 1.

EXERCISE 2.9

How could social media support your health promotion initiative?

health promotion interventions often come with a low risk of harm (compared to some clinical interventions, for example) the quality of evidence required may not need to be so great. Furthermore, it can also be difficult to provide information on the potential economic benefits, or return on investment (ROI). Therefore the evaluation needs to be planned at the same time as designing the initiative, and should include short-, medium- and long-term outcomes.

To estimate the possible ROI of an intervention in this scenario there is published information on ROI for contraception, including information published by the UK National Insititute for Health and Care Excellence (NICE) on the cost-benefits of long-acting reversible contraception. It is possible to model the savings of a 5%, 10% and 15% reduction in terminations in this age group. This, alongside the feedback from young people that school-based services and drop-in sessions with a regular health professional, will help to develop the business case for a new school-based drop-in service.

Using health promotion frameworks with this scenario

The Ottawa Charter for Health Promotion (WHO, 1986):

- Building healthy public policy: Work with schools, local authority and health providers to raise awareness of this important health and social issue.
- Creating a supportive environment: Work with schools to change PHSE lessons and the perception of teenage pregnancy. Provide teachers with essential information as well as the support of a health professional.
- Strengthening community action: Foster a culture of comprehensive sharing of information and support in developing personal resilience and relationship skills with young people. This can lead to a common understanding among young people and a culture where it is 'OK to ask'.
- Developing personal skills: PSHE lessons strengthened and nurse drop-in sessions made available for individual support.

- Re-orientating health services: School health nurse provision increased and scope of the nurse extended in targeted areas.

The health belief model:

- Perceived susceptibility: Local information shared on teenage conceptions and terminations, along with the statistical likelihood of getting pregnant following unprotected sex. Accompanying this, information shared on the safety of different forms of contraception and the impact of other risky behaviours on the likelihood of having unprotected sex.
- Perceived severity: Information provided on outcomes of teenage pregnancies for both the mother and baby.
- Perceived barriers: Ability to access support made easier.
- Perceived benefits: Discussed in PSHE sessions as part of group work.

Beattie's typology of health promotion model (Beattie, 1991):

- Negotiated individual: Young people empowered to make changes through increased relationship skills, knowledge and availability of support with regard to contraception choices.
- Negotiated collective: Within PSHE classes and group sessions, young people are provided with information to enable them to identify changes they can make.
- Authoritative collective: Content of PSHE classes changed.
- Authoritative individual: Support available from school health nurse to help individuals through stages of change.

FURTHER READING

Green J. 2000. The role of theory in evidence-based health promotion practice. Health Education Research 15(2), 125–129.

Lucas K, Lloyd B. 2005. *Health Promotion: Evidence and Experience*. Sage Publications, London.

Scriven A. 2010. *Promoting Health: A Practical Guide*. 6th ed. Elsevier.

Williams B, Bhaumik C, Brickell E. 2013. Lifecourse tracker, wave two report – Final. GfK NOP Social Research, London, England.

World Health Organisation (WHO). 2009. Milestones in health promotion: Statements from global conferences. http://www.who.int/healthpromotion/en/.

3

Healthcare public health

CHRISTOPHER CHISWELL, ROB F COOPER AND CHRIS PACKHAM

Introduction 45
Describing need 47
Responding to scarcity 48
Programme budgeting 50
Communicating effectively about scarcity 50
Interpreting data 51
Strategic decision making 52
SWOT analysis 54
PESTLE analysis 54
Structure of healthcare systems 58
Communication challenges in healthcare public health 59
Example scenarios 61
Further reading 65

PRE-READING

For an introduction to the theory covered in this chapter see Sections 3, 4 and 5 of Lewis G, Sheringham J, Lopez Bernal J and Crayford T, *Mastering Public Health: A Postgraduate Guide to Examinations and Revalidation*, 2nd ed., CRC Press, Boca Raton, FL, 2014.

INTRODUCTION

Healthcare public health, or population healthcare, seeks to optimise health and social care systems so that the combined effect on the care of individuals is to deliver maximum benefit to a whole population or society. It requires judgements on the benefits and costs of interventions, the quality and efficiency of services, the levels of resources and need, and the relative priorities of competing factors relevant to the population.

The delivery of healthcare services receives significant public and political interest, and the public health professional must be confident in communicating the principles and processes involved if services are to be, and perceived to be, equitable and effective. Healthcare public health can be practised within many different settings:

- Within local government authorities, local health boards or groups of clinicians acting as responsible bodies (e.g. local clinical commissioning groups in England), or in areas of joint commissioning or planning such as with mental health and social care.

- Within centralised, regional or grouped local bodies, acting above the local level and taking responsibility for system oversight, prioritisation and delivery of more complex and rare disease services, such as screening programmes.
- Within providers of services, ensuring that providers are able to pursue clinically effective and cost-effective, sustainable development and care models and to support clinicians across the interface with other organisations. Healthcare is typically provided in one or more of the following settings: (1) primary care, (2) secondary care, (3) tertiary care, (4) community services, (5) mental illness services, (6) child and maternity services, (7) elderly care services and (8) public health services (screening, health protection, health promotion etc).
- Within academic settings, to ensure that research recognises the constraints of health and social care delivery, ensuring recommendations and innovation are cost effective and can be appropriately weighted.

Practising public health tip 3.1 Working in and with healthcare organisations: Essential skills for the public health professional working with and within healthcare organisations include:

- Understanding the responsibilities of different organisations in healthcare and social care systems, and how interfaces between organisations operate and can be best managed.
- Critically assessing the strength and importance of evidence, and weigh it to reach a balanced judgement on its application.
- Applying the concept of health of populations rather than individuals, and the purpose of prioritisation in improving equity and value for money.
- Ensuring that prioritisation occurs (as resources are finite and possible healthcare interventions are potentially infinite) in a way that appropriately balances the utilitarian approach to public health with the importance of healthcare interventions to individuals as patients and their families.
- Conducting a timely analysis of data and other information sources, and presenting an analysis on the safety, quality and effectiveness of community- or hospital-based services. Often a pragmatic approach needs to be taken with regard to data analysis in order for it to be timely and useful. Very careful and detailed analyses that are produced too late are of little use.
- Making a pragmatic judgement as to how far to go with data finding, collection and analysis. It is often better to be 'approximately right' than 'precisely wrong'.
- Employing communication skills to interact with an array of professional and lay audiences, in both collaborative and hostile scenarios.

One of the most common challenges facing the healthcare public health professional is how to inform and influence the discourse that almost inevitably arises when need or expressed demand for healthcare exceeds a system's ability to supply services within a necessary financial allocation.

This 'scarcity' arises for several reasons:

- Changes in costs of healthcare and salaries of those providing care
- Direct costs of innovation and technological advances
- Survivorship, as people benefit from changes in life expectancy and treatments to live longer but may then suffer from chronic conditions for many years
- Changes in the funding provision for health services, or in a population's ability to fund their healthcare system
- Demographic change, and growth in certain segments of the population, particularly the 'older elderly' (see Figure 3.1)

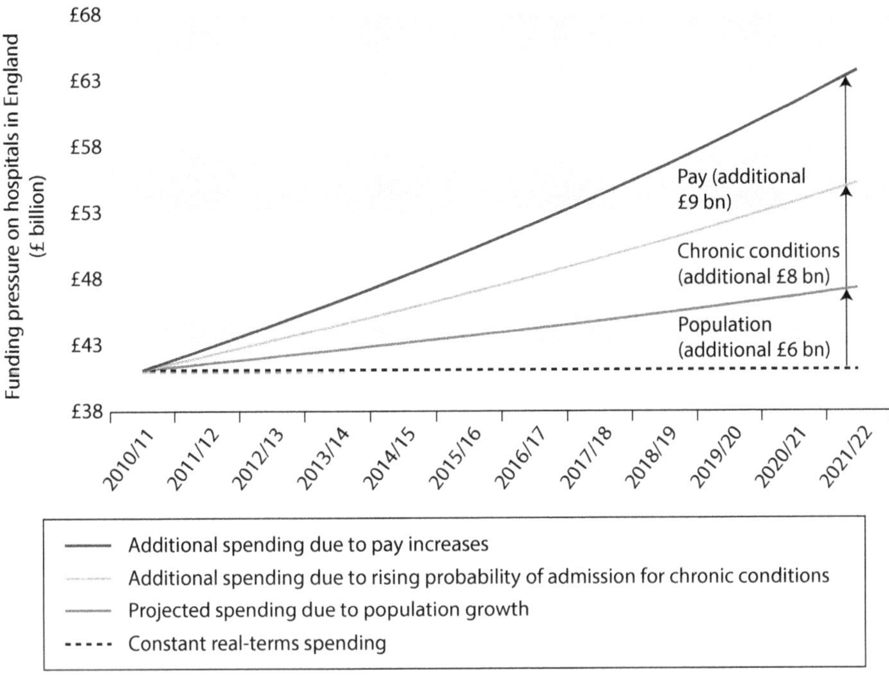

Figure 3.1 Funding pressures on acute services in England attributable to population change and to the rising probability of admission for chronic conditions. (From Roberts A et al. 2012. *A Decade of Austerity*, London: Nuffield Trust. With permission.)

- Increased demand for care and treatments, and rising expectations about the components of the service provided
- Priorities of a given society compared to the objective need of the individuals within that society
- Variation in the level of input required in different populations to achieve the same outputs

The effect of these variables is seen as a gap between what can be provided and what is required. For the National Health Service (NHS), this is most clearly seen in the funding gap that projections suggest will open between specified funding and pressures on services.

DESCRIBING NEED

Public health professionals should be familiar with Bradshaw (1972), which describes four types of need that emerge in health and social care settings: normative need (that which might be objectively identified for those in a system), felt need (perception of required care by members of a given system), expressed need (care or treatment that is requested of the system) and comparative need (requirements identified by comparing similar individuals within a system).

Health economics differentiates need from supply and demand, and it is helpful to review the work of Stevens and Gabby (1991) when being asked to consider these factors (see Figure 3.2).

Area 1: Unmet need for which there is no demand or supply

Area 2: Demand for which there is no supply (service) but there is no real need

Area 3: A service supplied which is neither wanted nor needed

Area 4: A service for which there is both a need and demand but inadequate provision of service

Area 5: A service which is wanted and provided but there is no real need

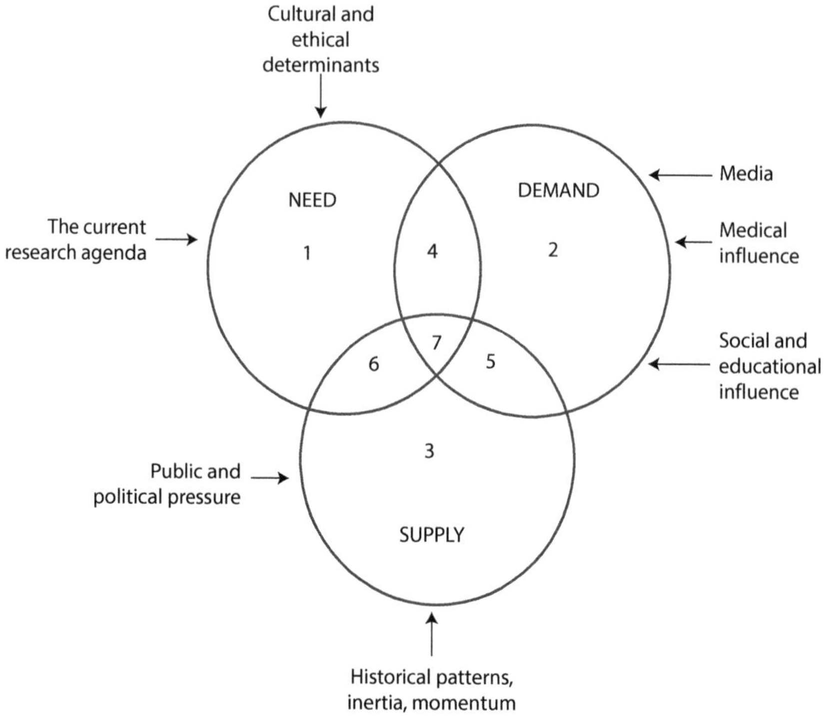

Cultural and ethical determinants

NEED

1

DEMAND

2

4

7

6

5

3

SUPPLY

Media

Medical influence

Social and educational influence

The current research agenda

Public and political pressure

Historical patterns, inertia, momentum

Figure 3.2 Overlaps and influences of need, supply and demand. (From Stevens A, Gabby, J. 1991. *Health Trends* 23(1), 20–23. With permission.)

Area 6: A service is needed and provided but uptake is poor as it is not utilised

Area 7: A service which is needed, provided and appropriately utilised

RESPONDING TO SCARCITY

Allocating resources within finite systems requires that a decision is made on what will be done and what will not be done. This process is called prioritisation. It should be recognised that not everyone readily accepts the need for prioritisation and intentionally refers to it instead as rationing in order to try to prevent it and its consequences from affecting their area of interest. It recognises that each decision to act consumes resources that will no longer be available for other competing needs or demands (opportunity cost). When weighing up the costs of such resource use, health economic principles should also be considered with regard to marginal costs and sensitivity analysis.

EXERCISE 3.1: Unmet needs and improving supply

Imagine a service such as community care for people with mental illness is identified by a health needs assessment as requiring expansion. Such a service may not be viewed by a provider as desirable for expansion and they may have concern about costs.

Consider how a provider could be asked to take on additional work – a public health professional should be able to ascertain what could be achieved at marginal cost and hence increase the likelihood of affordability.

This finite capacity to act means that attempting to make single decisions in series will be less successful than when a total set of options for a system are appraised in parallel. Each development will offer benefits, but it is only when we consider them together that we understand how many of them and what proportion can be delivered within the available resources. Knowing all the options means we can also make informed choices.

If we make single decisions as funding opportunities arise, we may find that all our resources are already committed when better investments later present themselves. Alternatively, we may fail to use resources effectively because we are holding excessive reserves.

It is recognised that as resources are finite, at least one of the following three factors has to be limited:

1. The time it takes to receive a service (manifests itself in 'waiting lists')
2. The number of people or proportion of a population eligible to receive a service (manifests itself in a multi-tier service)
3. The range of services available (manifests as a less than 'comprehensive' service)

EXERCISE 3.2: Explaining prioritisation

How would you explain the need to prioritise certain diseases and treatments to different stakeholders? For example, prioritising community care for people with dementia over other services to:

- A member of the public?
- A local politician?
- A hospital consultant/secondary care clinician?
- A primary care clinician?
- A journalist?

Healthcare systems need to have established processes for making these decisions. Effective prioritisation requires:

- A consistent approach so that there is a fair and open process, applied to the same standard across decisions
- An ethical framework, to help a set of decision makers understand the scope and principles of their decision making
- Clear understanding of the value of treatments, for example, the types of acceptable evidence, and econometric measures such as the quality-adjusted life year (QALY)
- An open mechanism by which the system can be held to account and challenged on grounds of fairness and reasonableness

Practising public health tip 3.2
Prioritisation: If rational and fair prioritisation is being opposed by the 'this is rationing' argument, be ready to explain that prioritisation still has to occur when total resources are being increased, so it is not only about reducing services (or making 'cuts').

An example of this in practice can be seen with the NHS Wales prioritisation and decision making framework, available from http://www.wales.nhs.uk. The framework gives NHS Wales an objective reference point in making decisions in the context of scarcity, setting out a standardised approach which they will take for all funding applications. There is also an explicit statement of the ethical principles underlying their decision making adapted from a common standard recommended by the UK Royal College of General Practitioners (Oswald and Cox, 2011):

> Aim to use limited resources to: Do as much good as possible whilst being fair. Doing as much good as possible means maximising health (and any other justifiable) benefit. Sometimes it may be justifiable to do less overall good in order to be fair (e.g. when targeting resources at a deprived group). When considering what is fair, in this guidance we argue that commissioners can apply two fundamental principles of human dignity: every person's life has intrinsic value and is worthy of equal concern; and autonomy: each of us has responsibility for the governance of our own life.

Many other similar responsible bodies operate within a similar framework.

EXERCISE 3.3: Explaining ethical frameworks

How would you explain to a member of the public why most ethical frameworks suggest that every individual is worthy of equal concern? For example, imagine being at a public consultation event where acute hospital services are being centralised from three or four local small hospitals onto one site. Increased efficiency and sustainability may benefit many individuals, but reduced ease of access may dis-benefit others.

PROGRAMME BUDGETING

Another example of a collective and comparative planning process is programme budgeting. The 'whole spend' for a disease or symptom grouping is calculated. It enables discussions between different areas ('should learning disabilities receive more investment than health visitors?') and within areas ('should we spend more on surgical procedures or preventative drugs for responding to patients with heart disease?').

Closely linked to this process is the need to understand the strength and reliability of evidence. Reaching this judgement requires assessment of the efficacy of the search strategy used to identify evidence, the research methods used, and the fair application of these methods to remove systematic error. It is useful to read 'How to Read a Paper: The Basics of Evidence Based Medicine' (Greenhalgh, 2014). Toolkits exist to support these assessments, and public health professionals should be familiar with levels of evidence and methods of appraisal.

Practising public health tip 3.3 Critical appraisal of evidence: When asked to comment on, or appraise, evidence papers, use a standardised toolkit wherever possible. This ensures you take a systematic approach and will give a common language to any further discussions about your assessment. The following may assist:

CASP: Critical Appraisal Skills Programme. Training and appraisal resources. Available from http://www.casp-uk.net/.

CEBM: Centre for Evidence Based Medicine. Blogs, resources and toolkits on appraisal. Available from http://www.cebm.net/.

GRADE: Grading of Recommendations Assessment, Development and Evaluation. Used by some major collaborations to prepare summary recommendations. Available from http://www.gradeworkinggroup.org/.

IDEAL: Idea, Development, Exploration, Assessment, Long-Term Follow-Up. An example of a specific tool for examining progress of developing a surgical intervention. Available from http://www.ideal-collaboration.net/.

EXERCISE 3.4: A health-related report in the media

Select an academic paper that has recently generated a significant media story (for example, around improvements in cancer survival or the effects of diet on health). Using one of the evidence toolkits, appraise the paper and then consider how you would respond to the article if you were asked for comment from a local journalist.

COMMUNICATING EFFECTIVELY ABOUT SCARCITY

When faced with scenarios that involve prioritisation or scarcity, the following checklist may be helpful in preparing a response:

1. Understand the audience and what their needs and agenda might be in the situation. Anticipate any emotional response or challenge to those in a leadership role (e.g. a call that 'the Board should resign!').

2. Use available resources to prepare a balanced argument, recognising the competing judgements that may be relevant.
3. Refresh your explanations of statistical or evidence statements you may be required to explain (e.g. clinical effectiveness, cost effectiveness, cost-benefit analysis, sensitivity analysis, significance).
4. Consider the best method to communicate your evaluation and decision, and what resources you might need if further investigation is required.

INTERPRETING DATA

Alongside the assessment of evidence, good decision making requires accurate interpretation of data into intelligence relevant to the decision or process.

EXERCISE 3.5: Information on health needs and healthcare evaluation

Before reading the 'Strategic Decision Making' section, write a list of the sources of information that you are aware of that might be relevant for undertaking a health needs assessment and/or a healthcare evaluation.

Data can originate from many sources:

- Surveys, questionnaires, censuses and feedback from patients – there are often routine national surveys of aspects of health (e.g. Health Survey for England) and feedback systems for quality of healthcare (e.g. friends and family test in England) which are based on the Net Promoter Score principle utilised by many healthcare systems worldwide.
- Routine data collections as part of service delivery in most health and social care systems (e.g. hospital episode statistics, primary care or general practice records) or business processes such as payment systems for services whether in one or more of a state-run system, independent healthcare system or insurance based system. Episodes are often categorised by similar expected resource use using case-mix analysis systems, e.g. HRGs in England (healthcare resource groups [HRGs] used for tariff-based pricing in parts of UK) or DRGs in parts of the U.S. healthcare system (diagnostic-related groups [DRGs] used for prospective reimbursement).
- Databases and monitoring schemes (Vascular Registry, British National Formulary Yellow Card Scheme).
- Research findings, journal articles and trial data (e.g. incidence studies, prevalence studies, drug trials).
- Interviews and consultation surveys with the public, patients and clinical teams.
- Data linkages and secondary use of data (including 'dashboard' type presentations or analyses of data are undertaken without any prior specific question in mind but instead to see if there are questions or issues that can be identified that may be worth pursuing further).

EXERCISE 3.6: A report on poor quality local healthcare

A review report has found poor quality of care and/or poor mortality outcomes at a hospital. Consider how a public health professional might balance the potential harm of a population still using it for its service as compared to not using it so risking some or all of its services to close. Consider issues such as verifying the data, using a longer time period before jumping to conclusions, the overall effect on health of losing local services if not used and possibly losing other services closely integrated or reliant on the service being questioned.

EXERCISE 3.7: Financial difficulties in a healthcare provider

When a healthcare organisation has financial difficulties, Boards, Chief Executives and Finance Directors may state one or more of the following as reasons:

- Increased clinical costs (e.g. staffing, drugs, procedures) have occurred beyond their control.
- The funding methodology applied to them is 'unfair', as their cases are more difficult/complex than are represented by the funding system and they are therefore being underpaid.
- They are having to treat (ever-increasing) numbers of certain groups of patients for which they do not receive funding.

Consider how a public health professional would investigate and handle this situation when advising a body with responsibility for this healthcare provider. Remember that one or more of the above may indeed be true. Consider how a public health professional could ascertain whether or not this is the case and what sources of expertise could be accessed.

Data may be presented to the public health professional in raw, tabular, graphical or text form. Public health professionals should have a clear system for interpreting data, but should be ready to flex this approach to the specific needs of a situation, particularly where time may be limited or the data is incomplete.

Practising public health tip 3.4 Seven Cs of data appraisal: When approaching data, the following seven Cs may be helpful in making a structured judgement about its reliability and accuracy (from http://www.mindtools.com):

- **Collection** – How, when, where and why was the data collected?
- **Capture** – Is this a sample or a population? Is it representative and unbiased, and is it sufficient to answer the question?
- **Coding** – How has the data been recorded? Does this introduce any problems?
- **Confidence** – Have the effects of chance been considered? What might their impact be?
- **Comment** – What does the data show? In a timed situation, focus on highlighting the relevant and important findings.
- **Confounding** – What other reasons might explain the observed dataset?
- **Conclusion** – What conclusions can be drawn from the presented data?

Practising public health tip 3.5 Case-mix analysis: Case-mix analysis systems allow healthcare providers, planners, commissioners and funders to see how patients vary by different clinical characteristics. It is important to know their main pros and cons:

- Pros – They aggregate cases into a meaningful number of types of case (usually only several hundred categories) which can be considered and discussed as opposed to an almost infinite number of possible permutations of main diagnoses, secondary diagnoses and procedures.
- Cons – They can be oversimplistic and the criticism levied that a particular healthcare organisation's cases are more difficult than is represented by the case-mix analysis system.

STRATEGIC DECISION MAKING

Healthcare public health professionals are often required to contribute to strategic development within an organisation or system. As well as utilising prioritisation skills, this also requires other key competencies:

- Communication and negotiation skills. Communication is a two-way process, and techniques of elicitation and knowledge transfer are as essential as presentation and explanation (see Chapter 1 for more on communication skills).
- Health intelligence gathering and data interpretation.
- Options appraisal.
- Stakeholder analysis. Effectively implementing policies or strategies relies on the actions of many different individuals and organisations. Stakeholder analysis can support the public health professional and their team to ensure effective action (Box 3.1).

BOX 3.1: An example of basic stakeholder analysis

Stakeholder analysis is the systematic analysis of the relationship of individuals, groups or organisations with the project or action being considered. It involves the following three steps:

1. Identifying how stakeholders, who are connected to the project, are affected by its implementation or have power to influence its delivery
2. Analysing their current attitude to and engagement with the project
3. Deciding on the ideal future position for each stakeholder and actions that can be taken to help achieve this

Scenario: Closing a failing semi-rural general practice and transferring patients to a nearby surgery.

Step 1: Stakeholder identification Using a table, and in dialogue with others, identify the stakeholders (Table 3.1). Describe why they are a stakeholder in the project, and identify their current position and level of involvement. Also identify your current relationship with this group.

Step 2: Stakeholder assessment Having identified all the stakeholders, it can often be helpful to place them into a grid, categorising them by their level of power and their level of interest in the project. Each quadrant on Figure 3.3 categorises stakeholders into a broad grouping which can then help the public health professional to begin to think about how to manage each relationship:

- High power and high interest: Engagement with these stakeholders is critical to the success of a project. They are interested in what is happening, and have significant ability to shape future direction. Their needs should be understood in detail, and they should be managed closely and attentively.
- High power and low interest: This group can seem irrelevant to a project, but due to their level of authority, can be disruptive if their needs are not met. Examples often include regulatory bodies, not directly involved, but which could prevent a project going ahead if it does not meet their prescribed standards and expectations.
- Low power and high interest: These stakeholders can consume substantial project time, as they will be highly engaged with project progress. However, their low power means they may not be able to significantly influence the path of the project. As such, the initial response should be to keep them informed of progress. This group can also be a valuable source of information about the project.
- Low power and low interest: Stakeholder mapping may identify individuals or groups who have some connection to the project, but are neither interested in the project nor significantly able to influence its delivery. To maximise resources, minimum resources should be invested in this sector, although the opinions of these stakeholders should still be monitored.

Stakeholder mapping is a dynamic process, and it should be kept updated as positions and power change.

Step 3: Stakeholder action planning

Stakeholder mapping not only helps the public health professional understand relationships affecting the project; it can also be used to support its implementation. This final stage places each of the important stakeholders into one of four categories, based on their current relationship to project progress. Each position is then strategically evaluated, and the ideal future state is identified. Action planning can then take place to identify what each stakeholder requires to shift their opinion to the desired category (Figure 3.4).

This tool can be particularly powerful when the relationships between stakeholders are also identified. In the example, the supportive hospital chief executive has been involved in discussions with the elected representative due to an existing relationship of trust. Notice as well that it may sometimes be necessary to seek to decrease the influence of certain stakeholders if their contribution is destabilizing a change process.

As well as stakeholder mapping, there are many other tools and methodologies which exist to support the public health professional in setting future strategy, including strengths, weaknesses, opportunities and threats (SWOT) and political, economic, socio-cultural, technological, legal, environmental (PESTLE) analyses. These can support the public health professional in understanding an organisation or policy context, and in planning how they communicate and influence action on key themes.

SWOT ANALYSIS

A SWOT analysis seeks to identify the strengths, weaknesses, opportunities and threats connected to a project. The strengths and weaknesses consider internal factors that relate to the organisation or body undertaking the work, and the opportunities and threats look outward to the environment within which the project will be delivered.

A practitioner preparing to brief a locally elected representative on the introduction of a new vaccination campaign might prepare a SWOT analysis to inform their discussion (Figure 3.5).

PESTLE ANALYSIS

A PESTLE analysis is another tool for the public health practitioner to analyse the external environment affecting a particular issue or project. PESTLE provides a helpful taxonomy to capture the complex and shifting melee of influences that can impact on a project:

- **Political**: Government structures and how they influence health. This can include policy setting, accountability and specific statements made by elected representatives and leaders.
- **Economic**: Availability of resources to fund care, from either central funding mechanisms or the economic climate within which individuals must resource their own healthcare.
- **Socio-cultural**: How groups and individuals are interacting with healthcare, and the prevailing opinions on how services should be delivered and used.
- **Technological**: Ways that innovation is changing what healthcare can be undertaken, and the mode and place of care where it is delivered.
- **Legal**: The regulatory environment within which care is delivered, and the statutory requirements on organisations.
- **Environmental**: Sustainability, as well as changes in the need and supply of healthcare due to epidemiological drive and economic conditions.

SWOT and PESTLE analyses form an important part of strategic planning in many NHS organisations, and detailed examples can often be identified in trust business plans (an example is from Oxford University Hospitals, which can be found through their website: www.ouh.nhs.uk).

Table 3.1 Outline of stakeholders and their involvement

Stakeholder	Connection to project	Current opinion	Current involvement	Resources, influence and power	Current relationship	Risk to project
Practice patients	Currently attend practice; will have to move to new practice if it is closed	Want practice kept open (most) but some may think move is acceptable	Small action group	Internet, social media, willingness to talk to local media	Ad hoc meetings with chair of action group	Increased media coverage; potential legal challenges
Other local residents	Not directly affected by project, but aware surgery may close	Neutral	None		Ad hoc communication through local newspaper	Would significantly slow progress if they opposed
Local MP	Has been contacted by local residents and action group	Opposed to any changes that will see a practice close in the area	Has contacted health decision-making body via letter	Political connections; strong voice in local media	None	Could provide significant challenge to process
Practice staff	Employment affected by closure, but aware of poor performance within practice	Eager for permanent solution, and think merging practices would improve care	Already been notified as at risk and offered employment within new structures' two members of staff are on the reconfiguration project group	Some employees are members of professional and union bodies; one member of staff has previously been a local councillor	Monthly briefings being sent to all staff, as well as opportunity for meetings as required	Potential increased costs if staff unwilling to move practices and choose to take redundancy offer

(*Continued*)

Table 3.1 (*Continued*) Outline of stakeholders and their involvement

Stakeholder	Connection to project	Current opinion	Current involvement	Resources, influence and power	Current relationship	Risk to project
Other general practitioner (GP) practices	May gain patients if practice closes; have been providing locum cover to practice	In favour of closure of the practice	Have received formal notification of project and submitted data for analysis of local need	Several general practitioners are members of local health decision-making body board	Communication via practice bulletins	Could stop project going ahead
Public transport provider	Currently provide services that stop outside practice	Neutral	None	None related to decision; can change bus routes	None	Minimal
Local hospital chief executive	Have raised several concerns about quality of care at practice	In favour of closure of the practice	Trust has written to health decision-making body raising concerns about quality of care at the practice	Well-respected organisation within community; senior clinicians at hospital involved in relevant professional groups	Informal conversation with a director at the trust on project progress	Likely to have significant influence on local public opinion about the project
National care inspectorate	Aware of concerns and awaiting action by local health decision-making body	Looking for improvement in standard of care; neutral on means of achieving this	Statutory reporting mechanisms	Can intervene in local processes if problems not resolved	Ongoing statutory connection	Can issue guidance that would block progress on project

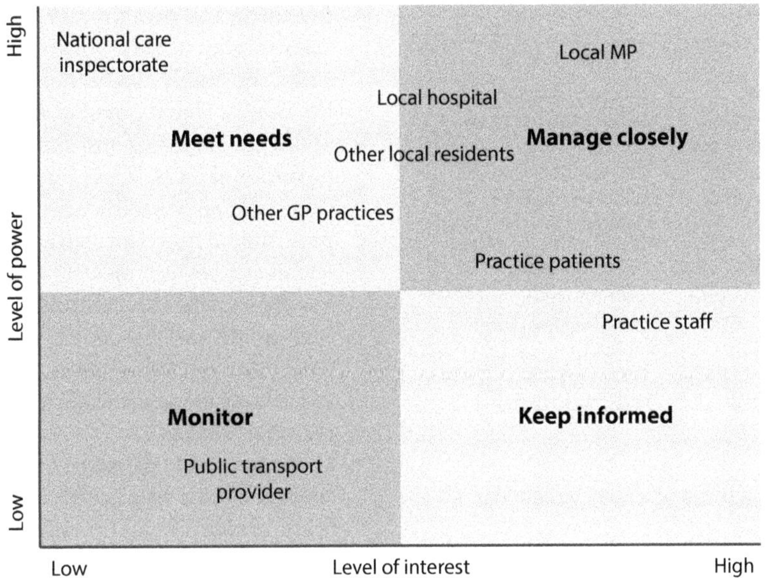

Figure 3.3 Stakeholder map.

Stakeholder	**Opposed**	**Permit**	**Assist**	**Enable**	**Action plan**
Practice patients		●	—	→	Need to explain reasons for change. Town hall event to be planned to explain case.
Local elected representative	●	→			Meeting set up with supportive local hospital director and elected representative to highlight safety concerns.
Local residents		●	→		Ongoing consultation exercise asking for views on how to improve local primary care services.
Practice staff		●			Continue to comply with processes for transfer of employment.
Other GP practices			←	●	Currently being perceived as a 'hostile takeover'. Discussion needed with local GP chair to ask for restraint in pushing debate.
Local hospital chief executive				●	Continue to keep informed. Asked to support conversations with local elected representatives.

Figure 3.4 The desired shift for each stakeholder when stakeholder action planning.

	Promoting	Inhibiting
Internal	**Strengths** • Vaccination will be available in all schools, giving universal coverage • Clear communications strategy already in place	**Weaknesses** • No central database to identify who has been vaccinated • Several schools have no dedicated room for vaccinations
External	**Opportunities** • Local celebrity endorsing campaign due to personal connection • Positive feature in local magazine about new campaign	**Threats** • National shortage of vaccine in next three months • Recent adverse reaction reported in national media

Figure 3.5 SWOT analysis of a new vaccination programme.

EXERCISE 3.8: SWOT and PESTLE analyses

Consider a project you are involved with or have encountered recently. Prepare a SWOT and PESTLE analysis, and identify how it could help you communicate the key messages to external stakeholders.

These approaches demonstrate how many decisions have positive and negative factors influencing them, and provide a structure to present a balanced view to decision makers.

STRUCTURE OF HEALTHCARE SYSTEMS

Healthcare systems are dynamic and frequently undergo re-organisation or re-structuring. However, there are common functions that are usually apparent within each system, and the healthcare public health professional will need to identify the influence and responsibility of each organisation to effectively deliver their duties.

Common responsibilities between many health systems include:

- **Planning and procurement at local level.** These bodies take responsibility for the sufficient supply of healthcare assets aimed at the needs of local populations.
- **Strategic planning and control at a sector or national level.** These high-level organisations take responsibility for the planning of provision of more specialised treatments, usually where volumes of care would be too low for local health commissioners to secure a high-quality service. Such bodies commonly determine screening policies and centres to evaluate evidence leading to national or regional policies.
- **Communicable disease control, environmental health and health improvement.** These systems focus on ensuring consistent and robust responses to infectious disease and environmental threats and on promoting interventions that improve the population's health, enhance disease prevention and reduce inequality. There is, in most countries, a government body/organisation responsible for delivering or advising on health protection services.
- **Regulatory functions, both professional and statutory.** These external regulators are given specific duties to assure the quality and stability of certain aspects of the health and social care system. These commonly include economic and financial regulation for health services, quality monitoring aiming to ensure care organisations provide and meet appropriate standards, and professional bodies having a responsibility to ensure that staff members working within health and social care are appropriately registered and safe to practise.
- **Integration organisations.** The complexity of health and social care structures means that bodies are needed to provide oversight and to ensure that different components work effectively together.
- **Patient champions and representatives.** Patients and members of the public need to have a strong voice in the planning and delivery of care, and many health systems have created specific structures to provide

this platform. Many third-sector organisations also contribute to this function. They can be disease specific (e.g. Alzheimer's disease organisations) or generic (e.g. patient associations).

- **Provider organisations.** These organisations provide healthcare and take responsibility for the delivery of care. They can be very large, delivering many different services, or much smaller and focused on one particular intervention or condition. Providers also need their own administration structures, and larger organisations will include a board of executive directors and non-executive directors, leading thousands of employees and undertaking a significant role in local communities and economies. Providers may be given responsibility for the provision of whole systems of care, and in these areas, they may act as commissioner of other organisations, as well as a direct provider of services.
- **Political oversight and accountability.** Although there is often a desire to separate healthcare services from political influence, the high public interest in having access to effective health and care systems, and the significant cost of health services to government, means that most political systems have a mechanism for oversight.

EXERCISE 3.9

Follow the link below to watch a video on NHS structures produced by The King's Fund which discusses the healthcare arrangement in England in 2013. Reflect on the complexity of the system and how each organisation performs the functions described above. As an example, consider which organisations you would need to influence to increase funding for managing increased winter demand on acute services in your local acute hospital.

http://www.kingsfund.org.uk/projects/nhs-65/alternative-guide-new-nhs-england

COMMUNICATION CHALLENGES IN HEALTHCARE PUBLIC HEALTH

Effective communication is a critical competency for the healthcare public professional. Success depends on the professional's ability to appraise and present information concisely, to handle uncertainty and conflicting opinions, and to quickly adapt their approach to their audience.

Table 3.2 provides a list of typical situations and key issues that may be encountered, and a framework for considering how communication can be enhanced.

Whatever the situation, communication will be more successful if the encounter is planned and considered in advance. For more detail on communication and listening skills, see Chapter 2. Specific themes to consider include:

- The purpose of the conversation from the point of view of the other stakeholders present. Consider the situation and motivation for the meeting or event. Use this to decide on the language and detail that may be required, and likely questions.
- Key information that needs to be conveyed. Building on the context of the conversation, identify salient information available to you, and explore key relationships in data or evidence that you may be required to discuss.
- How you can best structure the discussion. Having identified this information, sketch out themes or groupings that may help you structure your response. However, be ready to adapt or change as the situation develops or takes a different direction.
- Potential points of uncertainty or disagreement. If there are obvious gaps in knowledge or 'flashpoints' that you may be pressed to consider, plan an appropriate tone and comment for these areas.
- Critical explanations that you may require. Similarly, if there is a clear statistical value or concept you may be required to explain, make sure you have a concise, audience-appropriate definition ready.

Table 3.2 Communicating with stakeholders

Stakeholder	Possible situation	Key considerations	What success would look like
Public	Request for inquiry into quality of care at a local hospital (e.g. action group)	Understanding the specific concerns that need addressing Describing information in an accessible way, with no technical jargon Recognising there may be different views and handling this tension while still showing understanding	Member of the public has a clear understanding of the available information Principles by which a balanced decision can be made have been effectively shared and comprehension checked
Media	Interview on why a service is being rated poorly Interview on why a patient has been refused funding Interview on the expansion of a service or implementation of a new service	The topics of health service provision, rationing, and quality of care are highly sensitive A media scenario does not provide a format to convey high volumes of evidence Other organisations may be involved in the decision Handling the balance between a visible single patient and an unmet population need is challenging and consideration must be made for maintaining patient confidentiality unless they have consented to their details being used in the media	Clear, consistent, ethical principles with a strong emphasis on justice are highlighted as underpinning any resource allocation decisions The interviewee still has empathy and understanding of the complex and sometimes upsetting nature of the decisions being made Rights of patients to a fair consideration of their case are highlighted On occasions refusing to discuss or disclose individual patient information and so demonstrating the organisation's adherence to maintaining confidentiality
Health professional	Discussion on data relating to the quality of their service Investigation in to an adverse outcome	Conversation may be with someone who has expert subject knowledge beyond that of the public health professional There is a tension between 'my patient' and the needs of a service or population Discussion needs to be focused on evidence, but will often have to recognise the imperfections of available data	Health professional and public health professional have a shared understanding of the meaning of the data or evidence, and the reliability of the conclusion it suggests There is recognition of the principles around prioritisation and the ethical framework needed for these complex decisions
Politician	Briefing on reconfiguration of local health or social care services	Healthcare services can become strongly politicised issues and are very important to elected members	The importance of population health and equity in allocation of resources has been covered

(Continued)

Table 3.2 (*Continued*) Communicating with stakeholders

Stakeholder	Possible situation	Key considerations	What success would look like
	Discussion on quality of local healthcare services		The politician understands the salient points of any information presented
Organisation leader	Briefing on the performance of an organisation against a specific metric Impact of staff influenza vaccination rates on patient care (note overlap with other domains)	There is a growing expectation on senior leaders to have a comprehensive grasp of key issues at every level of their organisation e.g. 'Board to Ward' where on occasions they become carers.	The leader understands the critical issues and the implications of key findings or recommendations The leader is aware of any risks associated with the presented information and how this limits its relevance

EXAMPLE SCENARIOS

We will now introduce three examples to illustrate some of the points outlined above.

EXAMPLE 3.1: VARIATION IN SURGICAL PROCEDURE RATES

Variation in rates of a surgical procedure (on this occasion implantable cardiac defibrillators [ICDs] in seven areas of one UK region).

Scenario: You are asked to comment on the data to help brief a commissioning colleague who is worried about the variation in rates ahead of an important meeting.

Data presented: Table 3.3 shows the variation in new implants of ICDs in the region, 2014 and 2015, using directly standardised rates (DSRs) per million. Two specialist hospitals in the region carry out the surgery.

Table 3.3 Variation in new implants of ICDs by area in a region. Directly standardised rates (DSRs) per million population are shown for 2014 and 2015

Areas within the UK region	2014 (95% CI)	2015 (95% CI)
A	13 (4–22)	21 (12 30)
B	18 (3–33)	19 (2–36)
C	15 (1–29)	37 (28–46)
D	23 (10–36)	37 (26–48)
E	35 (29–41)	58 (45–71)
F	28 (0–56)	56 (35–77)
G	38 (22–54)	46 (32–60)
UK average	25 (21–29)	37 (32–42)
European average	63	63

Areas A–C refer to one surgical unit in one hospital.
Areas D–G refer to a different surgical unit in another hospital.

Questions asked

You may be asked by a person responsible for commissioning or planning health services:

- Regarding concern about the difference in the rate of ICD procedures by areas across the UK region. What does the data mean and what would we want to do next?
- What about trends over time?
- What are the main differences between areas?
- What is meant by directly standardised rates and why have they been used?
- How do confidence intervals (CIs) help in interpreting the data?

Possible answers

- These are directly standardised rates that allow direct comparison to be made between different age/sex structures in areas within the region.
- No area has achieved the European benchmark rate (63 implants per million), although the confidence intervals for two areas (E and F) do cover it in 2015.
- Confidence intervals should be mentioned but do not labour the definitional issues excessively.
- All areas have increased their rate between 2014 and 2015, but this change varies considerably between the areas. The UK increase between the two years is statistically significant.
- There are statistically significant differences between the highest rates (E) and lowest rates (A and B) but only in 2015; i.e. the gap has widened between the two years measured.
- Area E is significantly above and area A below the UK rate, but only in 2015.
- The variation in rates seems to reflect the known referral patterns to the two implanting hospitals; i.e. the rates are lower in A–C than in E–G.

Commentary

The questions for this section simply require you to summarise what the data is telling you. Basic public health science questions like CIs and standardised rates may be asked. Try thinking about all such basic epidemiological terms and practise describing them to your friends or family (see glossary for examples). It is harder than you think but is exactly what a public health professional may have to do in public health practice.

In this section, the material is healthcare related and therefore often quite clinical, but a detailed specialist knowledge of the exact clinical area is not essential. In the example given, it does not matter that the surgical technique relates to ICDs – it could relate to almost any procedure or diagnostic test – the principles will be the same.

EXAMPLE 3.2: MEDIA INTERVIEW ON THE IMPLEMENTATION OF A VASCULAR SURGICAL HUB

Scenario: You are being interviewed by a local news reporter on a current consultation to centralise surgery for major vascular (blood vessel) surgery to a single hospital site. This will involve this service no longer being provided at two other hospitals in the area.
Data presented: Three extracts taken from a local healthcare needs assessment.

1. **National recommendation** (adapted from report by National Vascular Society): It is no longer acceptable for emergency vascular care to be provided by generalist surgeons and radiologists who do not have a specialised experience. Commissioners are advised that abdominal aortic aneurysm (AAA) repair should only be undertaken in hospitals that perform at least 100 elective procedures over any 3-year period.

   Elective AAA repair should only be undertaken in hospitals where:

   a. There is a 24/7 on-call rota for vascular emergencies, with a vascular surgeon available overnight. Centres without 24/7 vascular cover should make immediate arrangements to transfer their elective and emergency arterial services to a local large-volume arterial hospital.

b. An on-site vascular laboratory is available.

2. **An extract of the activity of each hospital (Table 3.4).**
3. **Comment from surgeon leading the local multi-agency planning group:** 'The new national screening programme means that almost all of our patients have planned surgery and are well when they are admitted to hospital. Under the new system, we still plan to operate our outpatient clinics at all three sites, but the operations will all be undertaken at Hospital B'.

Table 3.4 Extract of activity data and assessment of local services

Hospital	Vascular operations per year	Vascular surgeon available overnight	On-site vascular laboratory
A	28	Yes	No
B	29	Yes	Yes
C	12	No	No

Questions asked

Common questions or concerns that might be raised in this scenario would focus on

- Concern that local people will have to travel further for services
- Increased risk to patients due to delays in treatment
- Questioning the motivation of the NHS for making these changes
- How the decision was reached

Possible answers

- Consistently focus on the quality and safety improvements for patients following the change.
- Communicate an accurate, lay-appropriate key message on mortality change, avoiding attempts to convey excessive statistical detail.
- Highlight that only the surgical episode will move and that other services will be maintained at other sites.
- Show empathy about the importance of local services, but consistent support for the agreed recommendations of the multi-agency planning group.
- Handle conflict by identifying areas of shared value and emphasising positives of the proposal.
- Signpost ways people can find out more about the proposal.

Commentary

This media scenario presents a different challenge to the more common health protection topics that may require interaction with a reporter. In this setting, there is likely to be a degree of challenge, and the public health professional needs to be clear on their core message around the motivation for the change. Appraisal of the scenario information should provide these key points, and any statistical information that is provided to support the conclusion should be simplified to provide appropriate sound bites during the interview.

Often, there are likely to be positives that strengthen the decision for a service reconfiguration, as well as 'burning platforms' that can be used to highlight why change is needed. In other resource allocation scenarios (for example, a decision about an individual funding request), the public health professional may need to describe why an organisation undertakes priority setting. Such explanations should be sensitive to the audience and the patients that may be affected.

EXAMPLE 3.3: BRIEFING ON OUTCOMES OF FRIENDS AND FAMILY TEST

Scenario: You have been contacted by the chair of the local health and wellbeing board. She has been reviewing the recent data release on the friends and family test for local maternity services. This is a routine feedback system along the principles of the Net Promoter Score for patients to simply report whether they would be happy for their friends or family to be treated in this organisation. She wants to discuss why all trusts are not achieving the same levels of positive feedback, and what you think could be done to improve the situation.
Data presented: Excerpt from friends and family test guidance from NHS England:

> All organisations providing NHS funded services will be using the friends and family test by April 2013 in all acute inpatient wards and emergency departments. From October 2013, the test will be extended to maternity services. Within 48 hours of receiving care or treatment, patients will be given the opportunity to answer the following question:
>
> *How likely are you to recommend our ward/emergency department to friends and family if they needed similar care or treatment?*

There are five possible answers from 'extremely likely' to 'extremely unlikely', as well as 'don't know'.

The friends and family test score is calculated by subtracting the proportion of people who answer either 'extremely unlikely', 'unlikely' or 'neither likely or unlikely' from the number who answer 'extremely likely'. Those who answer 'likely' or 'don't know' are not used as a numerator in either proportion. Table 3.5 shows the friends and family test data for your local hospitals providing maternity services.

Table 3.5 Friends and family test data for local hospitals

			Breakdown of responses						Mode of collection			
Name	**Total responses**	**Friends and family test score**	**Extremely likely**	**Likely**	**Neither**	**Unlikely**	**Extremely unlikely**	**Don't know**	**Text message**	**Kiosk**	**Paper based**	**Online survey**
Hospital A	2	100	2	0	0	0	0	0	0	0	2	0
Hospital B	126	83	106	17	2	0	0	1	7	0	119	0
Hospital C	25	73	16	6	0	0	0	3	0	0	24	1
Hospital D	83	70	58	23	1	0	0	1	0	0	83	0
Hospital E	218	66	146	62	1	2	2	5	0	0	218	0
Hospital F	56	57	37	14	2	3	0	0	56	0	0	0

Questions asked

Common questions that might be raised in this scenario would focus on:

- Why Hospital A is performing so strongly with a score of 100 compared to other trusts
- Whether the chair should take immediate action to address possible quality issues at Hospital F
- What factors might influence the presented data, and how could this be explored further
- How the accuracy of the test could be improved

Possible answers

- Clear, concise and simple explanation of the friends and family statistic. But if needed be able to go through an example i.e. the score for Hospital E is $(146 - 1 - 2 - 2) \times 100 \div (218 - 5) = 66$. Point out the 'likely' responses are excluded in this score and that its range is 0–100.
- Key elements highlighted from the presented data, including variation in the number of respondents and the methods of collection (Note that 95% of all responses were favourable and that Hospital A only had 2 respondents and Hospital F only received text responses)
- Discussion of wider system issues, including types and numbers of patients at different hospitals, and the potential for genuine differences in the quality of care at different sites
- A credible and pragmatic plan for further investigation of the issues highlighted, with identification of key organisations and additional relevant data sources

Commentary

This scenario challenges the public health professional to grasp a statistic they may not be immediately familiar with and make recommendations on variation in practice. It is unlikely that the chair of the health and wellbeing board will be hostile as they are keen that high quality services are provided, but they may be seeking to take direct action where further investigation would be a more appropriate first step. The public health professional must guide this conversation, highlighting issues of data quality and the potential range of reasons for variation. However, they must also not defend what may potentially be an early warning sign of failing care. Success in this scenario would be agreement on an action plan for further investigations, and the chair feeling suitably briefed with a clear understanding of the statistic and the local data.

FURTHER READING

Austin D. 2007. Priority setting: An overview. NHS Confederation. http://www.nhsconfed.org/Publications/Pages/Prioritysettingoverview.aspx.

Daniels N, Sabin J. 2002. *Setting Limits Fairly: Can We Learn to Share Medical Resources?* 1st ed. Oxford: Oxford University Press.

Department for Communities Local Government. 2009. Multi criteria analysis manual for making government policy. https://www.gov.uk/government/publications/multi-criteria-analysis-manual-for-making-government-policy.

Fisher R, Uri W. 2012. *Getting to Yes: Negotiating an Agreement without Giving In.* London: Random House Business.

Gigerenzer G, Gray M. 2013. *Better Doctors, Better Patients, Better Decisions.* 1st ed. Cambridge, MA: MIT Press.

Greenhalgh T. 2014. *How to Read a Paper: The Basics of Evidence Based Medicine.* 5th ed. London: Wiley-Blackwell.

Setting priorities in health. 2011. Nuffield Trust. http://www.nuffieldtrust.org.uk.

Subscribe to the healthcare public health newsletter. www.healthcarepublichealth.net.

Whittington R, Johnson G, Scholes K. 2010. *Exploring Strategy.* 9th ed. London: Prentice Hall/Financial Times.

4

Leadership and change management

RACHAEL LESLIE AND ADAM TURNER

Introduction 67
A brief history of leadership and management 68
Leadership styles 68
Public health leadership context: Using the healthcare leadership model 71
Understanding yourself as a leader 71
Managing change 73
Importance of motivation 77
How we react to change 77
Influencing people 79
Emotional intelligence 80
Application in your role 81
Preparing for a meeting 81
Understanding current public health priorities and policies 82
Project management 83
Successful partnership working 83
Further reading 86

PRE-READING

- A general introduction to leadership and change management can be found in Section 5 of Lewis G, Sheringham J, Lopez Bernal J, and Crayford T, *Mastering Public Health: A Postgraduate Guide to Examinations and Revalidation*, 2nd ed., CRC Press, Boca Raton, FL, 2014.
- Leadership advice and information with a National Health Service (NHS) focus, http://www.leadershipacademy.nhs.uk/resources/oc, and with a local government focus, http://www.localleadership.gov.uk/.

INTRODUCTION

Clear communication is the most important element to successful leadership and this chapter will help you understand your role as a leader and how, from within this role, you can maximise your communication skills.

The career of a public health professional can begin from a range of backgrounds: clinical, healthcare, academic, community development and the voluntary sector. Some of your colleagues may have formally learned leadership and management skills, whereas others will have developed and honed these skills through delivering projects, working in teams and experiencing changes to the health economy around them.

Leadership is important at all levels of an organisation. It is not just the chief executive who uses leadership skills to manage change, influence people and work across organisations; public health professionals at all levels also use these skills in their daily roles. The theory and methods of analysing leadership provide practical tools to support individuals, teams and organisations to recognise, understand, evaluate and improve different elements of their leadership styles to improve their effectiveness.

This chapter has been developed to support public health professionals to understand the wider context of leadership within a public health role. It provides a background of leadership models and then covers contemporary thinking around systems leadership. This will help the modern-day public health professional operate successfully across boundaries within new health and care landscapes.

Concepts and practical examples are presented around managing change, influencing people and partnership working. These key areas will provide you with practical ideas to be successful within your leadership roles.

A BRIEF HISTORY OF LEADERSHIP AND MANAGEMENT

Although you can argue that the world has never been without it, contemporary leadership and management theory dates back to the early 1900s when Fredrick Taylor (1911) proposed the theory of scientific management and Henry Fayol proposed the functions of management. Both theories arose from the point of view that organisations were similar to machines in that leaders would command followers who all had specific tasks. Based on the assumption that the workplace is highly structured, there was little room for innovation and flexibility within the command and control environment.

Although somewhat before his time, Mayo in the 1930s began to develop human relations theory, which identified that people were not simply cogs in larger machines, but all motivated by different things, and good leaders need to understand the motivations of individuals to bring out the best in their workforce and increase productivity. It was not until the 1960s that this theory really began to be championed by Frederick Herzberg, who identified that we are all motivated by different things. Henry Mintzberg (1975) began to rationalise that managers and leaders needed to be able to flex between different roles. These could range from more scientific and structural roles focused on information processing through to managing relationships.

In the 1960s Douglas McGregor identified the concept of theory X and theory Y management to consolidate these dichotomies. Theory X managers assume that employees cannot be trusted to do their work and they need a strong element of command and control to achieve tasks. Theory Y managers assume that work is natural to people; we are motivated to do a good job, seek satisfaction in work and need little supervision.

The ideas above bring us to exploring the difference between management and leadership. Contemporary thinking has begun to acknowledge that there are strong differences between leadership and management, which is contextualised in the following quote:

> Managers do things right, leaders do the right thing. (Bennis and Nanus, 1985)

Table 4.1 allows you to start to explore the difference.

LEADERSHIP STYLES

Working in public health means working with a varicty of different stakeholders that will have different leadership styles at both the organisational and the individual level. Some of the more recognised styles are outlined below.

- *Trait theory:* Although not a leadership style, this represents the oldest way of thinking about effective leadership by focusing on identifying the personality traits of successful leaders. This encourages the perception that 'good leaders are born, not made' and that effective leaders

Table 4.1 Differences between managers and leaders

Managers	Leaders
Do things right	Do the right thing
Plan and make things happen within their system or remit	Deal with change across a system
React to need	Proactively seek out opportunity
Follow direction	Provide vision and future focus
Control and instruct people and resources	Motivate and coach people, bringing out the best in them through trust
Coordinate people's efforts	Inspire and energise effort
Enforce rules	Challenge and change rules

cannot be developed or taught. Contemporary thinking would argue with this, as it does not allow for the potential that we as human beings can grow and learn.

- *Transactional leadership:* The transactional leader causes followers to undertake tasks or achieve goals in return for something the follower wants – this may be pay, kudos or promotion. Transactional leadership considers how leaders should reward (and punish) their followers based on performance and results. Leaders and their teams achieve goals together, following the direction of the leader who effectively maintains power. Some may call this an autocratic leadership style.
- *Authoritarian leadership:* Similar to and sometimes referred to as an autocratic style, this is where leaders spell out the goals, deadlines and methods while making decisions on their own without any significant consultation with others. Here, the leader doesn't usually get involved in the group's work. Not surprisingly, researchers have found that you are less likely to see creative decisions under this style of leadership. However, it is a decisive way of leading and can suit high-risk, short-timescale decisions – the kind that surgical teams and fire crews have to take. The psychologist Kurt Lewin noted that leaders who adopt this style can go too far and be seen by others as overcontrolling and dictatorial. He also noticed that they often find it hard to move to a participative style – in other words, they get stuck in one mode of behaviour.
- *Transformational leadership:* A transformational leader could be considered 'the light in the darkness'. The transformational leader understands and taps into the values and motivations of followers to inspire them to achieve a common purpose. Transformational leaders often have strong vision and appeal that they use to raise the conviction and confidence of followers. Such leaders are highly visible and engaging, possess a great deal of emotional intelligence and self-awareness, and encourage and motivate employees' productivity through inspiring a shared purpose toward a shared vision of the future. They trust their followers to help them achieve the overall vision by working together toward it.
- *Delegative leadership:* Lewin classes this as a leadership style, but some may feel it is non-leadership. The delegative style means the leader hands over responsibility to the group. He or she lets them set goals, decide on work methods, define individuals' roles and set their own pace of work. It is very much a hands-off approach. It can work well provided the group shares the same overall intent and direction as the leader and if he or she trusts all members of the group. However, there is always a risk that individuals may become dissatisfied with either their roles or the group's goals, and therefore lose motivation.
- *Functional leadership:* This focuses on the action areas that a leader must address to be effective and the behaviours needed to achieve these. One of the most contemporary and widely used models is the action-centred leadership model developed by Adair (1973), which proposes that good leaders will consider the task at hand, the team's role in making the task reach fruition, and also how to enable the individual to support the team in achieving the task.

- *Participative leadership:* Sometimes called democratic leadership, this style requires input from the entire team, and although the final decision may rest with the leader, they will demonstrate how the group has led and influenced the decision that is made through a highly engaging process. It is good for achieving longer-term change, as followers help co-create the future and therefore are more likely to believe the vision. One weakness is that this style can struggle to create rapid change.
- *Servant:* This style of leadership considers that the leader must put the needs of their followers first, and that happy followers mean they will work toward achieving the end vision. This style can have issues with balancing the needs of followers against needs of the business and its stakeholders.
- *Situational leadership:* Contextualised by Hersey and Blanchard (1977), situational leadership is a more contemporary way of looking at leadership based on the idea that the leader's behaviour, and how they deal with any given situation, should vary according to the circumstances they are facing. In essence, it acknowledges that all leadership styles can be valid at different points of time in different situations. For example, when responding to an emergency, authoritarian leadership is required, whereas transformational leadership may be better suited if the goal were to develop a new model of working.
- *Systems leadership:* At the time of writing, this form of leadership is particularly relevant to public health in England. The role of public health teams in England now spans across health, social care and local government functions, and to be successful it requires multiple stakeholders to work together for the greater good of the public. These attributes form the basis of systems leadership: to work both across boundaries and collaboratively for the greater good.

A contemporary definition of systems leadership is

> an attempt to effect change for the social good across multiple interacting and intersecting systems, resting on the assumption that better and more efficient public services can result from more joined-up working across multiple service sectors. (Ghate et al., 2013)

From Ghate et al.'s (2013) review of systems leadership the following areas were identified to enable systems leadership (these are particularly important to consider in the context of any public health leader who is wishing to strategically align public health activity across multiple systems):

- Use influence, not formal power.
- Align around a common vision or purpose.
- Focus on outcomes and results, not processes.
- Have strong but robust and honest relationships.
- Connect political and organisational leadership.
- Create a focus for individual accountability and 'felt responsibility'.

EXERCISE 4.1: How does this relate to you?

Considering the above, try answering the following:

What leadership style appeals to you most? Why?	What leadership style is predominant in your team? Is it the most effective?	What leadership style do you think is most important to you as you grow as a public health leader?

Practising public health tip 4.1 Leadership styles: Recognising and adapting to different leadership styles in different scenarios will help you to facilitate a successful outcome. It is often quite straightforward to observe and identify other people's leadership style. Also it might be useful to ask them directly what their leadership style is and what style they prefer. Understanding the preferred approach of the person you are working with will help you to understand their behaviours and actions.

PUBLIC HEALTH LEADERSHIP CONTEXT: USING THE HEALTHCARE LEADERSHIP MODEL

The NHS in England has developed a long-established approach to defining contemporary leadership competencies that enable healthcare leaders to perform at their best. This approach will also be useful for public health practitioners and specialists working in local government authorities or other organisations. Originally, the NHS developed a leadership qualities framework which defined the key behavioural competencies any leader should be able to demonstrate to be successful. Over time, wider versions were developed including medical and clinical versions of this framework. Recently, it was identified that previous iterations of this framework were redundant, as healthcare is rapidly changing, and a model was needed that was dynamic and could reflect this.

The NHS Leadership Academy began the development of what has become known as the Healthcare Leadership Model (2013) by reviewing contemporary academic literature and conducting behavioural interviews with a wide variety of leaders from diverse backgrounds across healthcare. The resultant model identified the following key leadership domains relating to personal qualities:

- Inspiring shared purpose
- Leading with care
- Evaluating information
- Connecting our service
- Sharing the vision
- Engaging the team
- Holding to account
- Developing capability
- Influencing for results

Leaders within healthcare are able to assess themselves against these domains by using a self-assessment tool.

For more information visit the Healthcare Leadership Model website: http://www.leadershipacademy.nhs.uk/resources/healthcare-leadership-model/

UNDERSTANDING YOURSELF AS A LEADER

Methods for understanding your leadership style and its impact on others include the following.

Myers-Briggs Type Indicator (MBTI)

MBTI is a popular tool for helping individuals to understand their preferred leadership style and associated strengths and weaknesses by using a psychometric questionnaire. The process involves answering a series of questions resulting in being provided with a summary of your personality type representing four pairs of traits:

- Extraversion (E) or introversion (I)
- Sensing (S) or intuition (N)
- Thinking (T) or feeling (F)
- Judging (J) or perceiving (P)

People are identified with one of each pair of traits (e.g. ENTP) giving a total of 16 personality types. A description of the types and information about how to access the tool can be found here: http://www.myersbriggs.org/my-mbti-personality-type.

360° feedback/multi-source feedback (MSF)

360° feedback (also known as multi-source feedback [MSF]) is a tool to help individuals identify

EXERCISE 4.2: Myers-Briggs

Of the 16 Myers-Briggs Types, which one are you? Think about the teams you work in and the types of people in those teams. How does your personality type complement other members of the team? Could this knowledge help you communicate with colleagues – for example, by focusing on what others find interesting or rewarding? How does your personality preference relate to your colleagues?

If you get a chance, we highly recommend that you undertake a formal MBTI assessment, or similar personality profiling tool as part of your leadership development with a trained facilitator. More information on MBTI can be found at www.opp.com/en/tools/MBTI or an alternative free-to-access profiling tool based on similar personality preference theory by famous psychologist Carl Jung can be found at www.16personalities.com.

what their leadership strengths and development needs are. The process includes getting confidential feedback from line managers, peers and direct reports. As a result, it gives an individual an insight into other people's perceptions of their leadership abilities and behaviour.

Your organisation may have a tool and process for undertaking 360 reviews. Otherwise the NHS Leadership Academy provides a tool. For a small fee, the model allows for 360° feedback, allowing participants to invite managers, peers, staff they line manage and wider participants to rate their behaviours against each of the elements within the key leadership domains. This can then help the user to reflect on how they perceive themselves and how others perceive them; this can enable deep learning into their own leadership style and any development needs arising from this.

More information on this model and how you can participate in self-assessment for 360° feedback can be found at the NHS Leadership Academy website: http://www.leadershipacademy.nhs.uk.

EXERCISE 4.3: 360° review

Carry out a 360° review. First predict how you think people will answer in general. Then break down the responses you get to:

- Peers
- Those who report to you
- Those you report to

Examining the difference between how you perceive yourself and how others perceive you may prove constructive and provide areas to improve your communication skills. Additionally, identifying differences between how people at various levels in the organisation view you should again give you valuable insight into how you interact with people.

EXERCISE 4.4: From the description of leadership styles above and after undertaking a Myers-Briggs/360° review

- Which style best describes your natural approach?
- What style would you like from an immediate line manager?
- What style would you like from the leader of an organisation you would like to work in?
- What style of leader would you like in an emergency situation?
- What style of leader would you like when designing a new service?

Methods for developing your leadership style

- *Formal leadership programmes:* There are likely to be a variety of leadership development programmes available to you through your employer, and as part of your development it is suggested that you contact your local learning and development department to support and signpost you to the best programme for you.

- *Mentoring and coaching:* The benefits of mentoring and coaching are to support you to develop both your professional and leadership skills. Successful leaders will know who to go to in order to provide them with advice and support, and also actively utilise a coach to help them identify and achieve personal goals. It can be difficult to understand the differences between mentoring and coaching so these have been highlighted in Table 4.2.
- *Personal development plan (PDP):* Write a PDP during your appraisal to identify areas of learning and skills that you would like to develop. These can relate to your current role or future desired roles, and can also be an opportunity to develop your learning in an area of personal interest.
- *Action learning sets (ALSs):* ALSs are usually informal groups of peers that meet to discuss issues and provide support for each other. They can be facilitated. Groups may meet quarterly or monthly to discuss a challenge or issue that a member of the group is facing. Other members of the group are then invited to provide perspectives, support and advice.

  ALSs may also be set up to tackle specific challenges as a group and can be effective for particular learning styles. For example, a group may be established to prepare for an exam and may use regular sessions to practice exam questions with each other and share answers and approaches.

MANAGING CHANGE

Overview of managing change

Managing change is a fundamental part of any public health leader's role. After all, the impact of public health leadership decisions will directly impact upon the long-term health and wellbeing of our population. In fact, change management forms part of all health and care professionals' roles as our field is continually advancing in both theory and practice, and how our practice is managed and governed.

One of the most radical changes seen to public health in the UK arose from the Health and Social Care Act (2012), which removed public health from its more traditionally rooted health foundations and placed the profession within the remit of the local government authority, producing a national body, Public Health England, to manage the profession. For our purposes, we can consider a simple definition of change management as

> an approach to transitioning individuals, teams, and organizations to a desired future state. (Kotter, 2011)

Table 4.2 Differences between mentoring and coaching

Mentoring	Coaching
• Developing you as a professional/expert	• Wider general personal and leadership development focus
• A mentor is usually an expert in the area you wish to become more skilled within, imparting their knowledge and experience onto the individual	• A coach does not have to be an expert in the individual's work area, but uses skills to identify solutions to individual challenges
• More informal meetings, ad hoc support and less structured	• Formal and structured meetings with a goal focus
• Long-term relationship	• Short-term relationship, usually between 3 and 6 focused meetings
• Focus on career and professional development	• Focus on achieving developmental goals or solutions to a work-based challenge

Using change models

There are many models that consider change management. Here, we will provide several models of various complexities that will help you, as a leader, contextualise change management.

GAP ANALYSIS

When we consider our role as leaders of change, the simple gap analysis analogy is often the easiest place to start. The model asks you, as a leader or as a team, to consider and analyse the current state of affairs. It then asks you to consider the future, what you want it to be like, your vision, and what you want to achieve. The key part to this simple model is to ask yourself how you intend to get there. This will give you a variety of actions that you need to undertake to make your change a reality (Figure 4.1).

It is also worth thoroughly exploring the potential impact of the changes you propose to make before you fully decide upon them – will they really get you to your future vision? By taking this approach, you will be able to identify all of the actions that you need to take to reach your vision.

THREE STAGES OF CHANGE

The psychologist Kurt Lewin (1947) proposed a simple three-step model of change. Building upon gap analysis, it can be likened to how water can move states between being ice and liquid and back again (Figure 4.2).

1. *Un-freeze:* Start the process to make your change and understand what's driving things to change shape. What does the future look like? Why should you go there? What is the evidence for this? What are the implications? How will you address challenges?
2. *Change:* Create movement toward your intended change. How will you shape it? Your situation is now in a phase of re-shaping and movement where everything you do should be moving you one step closer to your future vision. How are you engaging people and selling the vision? Who is helping you get there? How are you overcoming obstacles? What are your milestones? Is the future vision still the same shape you first intended it to be? Change doesn't happen overnight, and it may take some time before your melted ice cube has reached the shape that you need it to.
3. *Re-freeze:* At this point, we can assume you have reached your desired shape, or rather, your future vision. This phase is called re-freezing as it implies when we reach our goals, the change is no longer a change, but rather it becomes business as normal. At this point it is really important to celebrate the success of your

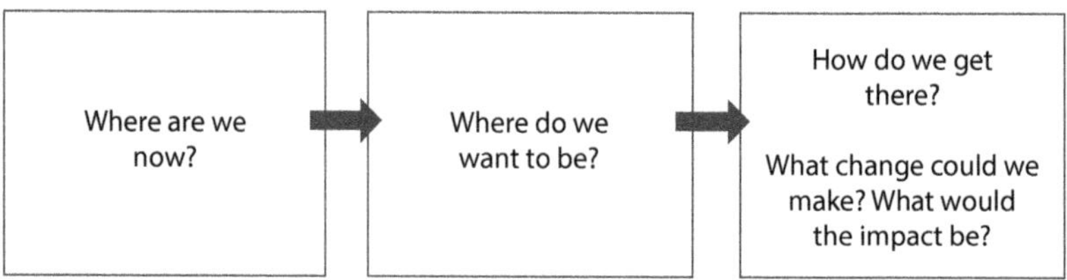

Figure 4.1 Gap analysis model.

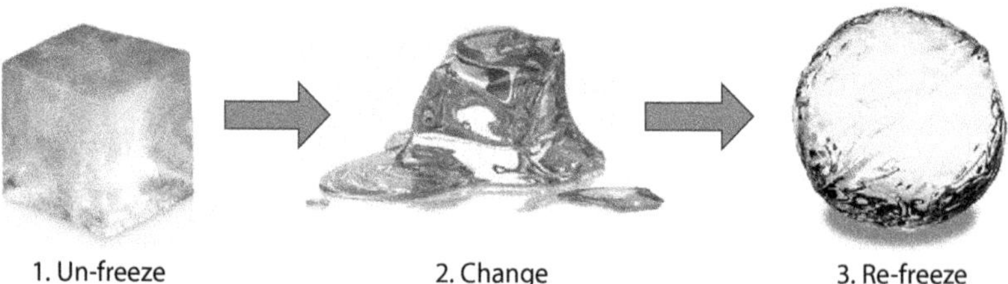

Figure 4.2 Three-stage change model. (Adapted from Lewin K. 1947. *Human Relations* 1, 5–41.)

change and recognise and reward the people who helped you get there. It's also important to consider whether this will be a long-term change – have you really done everything you can to embed it within your culture?

Although highly regarded, some criticism of Lewin's model is how it implies we can simply re-freeze and continue in a world where we don't have to change. Within health and social care, we know that the one constant is change. For most current professionals, there possibly has never been a time when we were not in some form of change or transition period.

It may therefore be more useful to consider the world around you as a constantly changing ice sculpture. You may need to continually shape and re-shape what you are trying to achieve. At one point you may wish to re-shape one element, and at another time you may wish to melt your entire sculpture and re-shape it completely.

FORCE FIELD ANALYSIS

During the same period Lewin also developed force field analysis. This looks at all of the factors (forces) for (helping forces) and against (hindering forces) your decision or change. Putting a score to these factors may help you decide whether or not to go ahead with a proposal or whether further work is needed before proceeding.

For instance, in the example below (Figure 4.3) it may be decided that the hindering forces are presently too strong and more work needs to be carried out to influence the existing factors, or introduce new factors, so that the helping forces 'win'.

EXERCISE 4.5: Think of a problem in your current job and apply force field analysis

- List all the helping and hindering forces (ideally with colleagues so a comprehensive list is generated).
- Score all the issues and see which force is the greatest.
- Think of ways you could improve the scores (either by introducing new forces or changing the influence of existing forces).

KOTTER'S EIGHT-STEP MODEL

Likened to Lewin's three-step model of change, Kotter (1995) developed an eight-step change model to help leaders conceptualise the process of change management. It centres around three phases: creating the climate for change, engaging and enabling the organisation, and implementing and sustaining for change (Figure 4.4).

Phase 1. Create the climate for change

Step 1. Create urgency: For a change to happen, people need to see that there is a need. As a leader, you will need to engage and convince your followers that the change is needed and

Helping forces	Weighting High (10)/Medium (5)/Low (1)	
Oral health assessment: Dental caries prevalence	High	10
Evidence base: Safety, dental health	Medium	5
Reduction in health inequalites	Low	3
	Total	**18 points**

Change: introduction of fluoridation in an area

Hindering forces	Weighting High (10)/Medium (5)/Low (1)	
Cost of implementation	High	10
Public protest groups: concerns about safety	Medium	5
Need to get agreement across multiple areas	Medium	5
	Total	**20 points**

Figure 4.3 Force field analysis of fluoridation decision.

Implementing and sustaining for change	8 – Make it stick
	7 – Build on the change
Engaging and enabling the organisation	6 – Create quick wins
	5 – Empower action
	4 – Communicate the vision
Creating the climate for change	3 – Create a vision for change
	2 – Form a powerful coalition
	1 – Create urgency

Figure 4.4 Kotter's eight-step model. (Adapted from Kotter J. 1995. *Leading Change*. Boston: Harvard Business Review Press.)

that it is a good thing. Your role is not only to provide a compelling argument backed up by evidence, but to engage followers in sharing your vision. At this point, don't just seek out the views of those who support your vision; a good leader will listen carefully to the views of those who don't necessarily agree with their vision as a useful critique and respond appropriately. Furthermore, how will you appeal to the values, hearts and minds of your followers? All of this will potentially lead to you identifying your coalition of change champions.

Step 2. Form a powerful coalition: Once you have identified your change champions who see the need for and support your vision, you need to work as a team to build momentum. It's important to utilise the ideas and value-added perspectives from your group. Their views will help shape and enhance your vision, thus creating a shared vision that has an emotional commitment from your followers; they become vested in your vision and will want to help you see it through to reality. How can these followers help you to continue to gain momentum?

Step 3. Create a vision for change: If your vision is too complicated, it will be difficult for others to follow and may fail to continue to gain momentum. At this point you should consider how you begin developing the narrative or strategy to explain your proposed change. A simple, compelling and clear vision will help everyone to understand what you are trying to achieve, no matter their personal view on your proposed change.

Phase 2. Engaging and enabling the organisation

Step 4. Communicate the vision: How can you bring your vision to life? It's not as simple as communicating it to people and telling them what to do. Why should they listen to you? What's in it for them? How will you address people's concerns and anxieties? You will also need to 'walk the talk' to ensure that everyone sees you role-modelling what you are trying to achieve. We can all say things, but it's our actions that will speak for themselves.

Step 5. Empower action: At this point you will have gained significant momentum and have recruited change champions to help progress your vision. However, how are you addressing the challengers and blockers? If left unaddressed, these elements could prevent your vision from becoming a reality. Blockers could be in the form of people who resist your vision or they could be physical, such as the resources aren't readily available; it could also be that there are unexpected developments that you hadn't accounted for that may impact on your progress. How are you going to manage these challenges? Don't avoid tackling them!

Step 6. Create short-term wins: The end product of your vision could be way off into the future. How will you keep motivated until then? Break up your vision into key milestones that are achievable in shorter time frames. This way, both you and your change champions will keep motivated as you incrementally progress toward your ultimate vision.

Phase 3. Implementing and sustaining for change

Step 7. Build on the change: Kotter takes the view that change projects fail in the longer term because they will state that they have reached their vision prematurely. Have you achieved long-lasting change, or is it more of a nominal number of quick wins? With every milestone you achieve, analyse it to consider the impact it is having. Do you have to adapt or change some of your future plans? Has your ultimate vision had to shift to make for a better end product? A key element for any leader of change is being able to have the flexibility to adapt their vision when the need arises, building upon the learning with each milestone along the way, and at the same time testing out how deeply rooted the impact of their changes really are. Discuss and share progress with your followers, recognise efforts made and reward them, and empower others to lead wider aspects of your vision.

Step 8. Make it stick: A change has been successful when it is seen to be business as usual and part of the culture you are working in. It stops being seen as a vision, and instead becomes part of your day-to-day work. Have you really reached your vision, or is there still some work to do?

NHS CHANGE MODEL

The NHS change model (NHS Improving Quality, 2013) is a contemporary model for leaders and practitioners to consider how to make a change become reality. The model and its elements can be useful for public health practitioners working in the NHS, local government or other organisations, particularly when working with partners and across departments and organisations (Figure 4.5).

Recognising that change is dynamic and ongoing, the model provides several domains that should be considered in order to drive toward successful change. Central to this model is the need for a shared purpose and that for the change to be successful, all members of the NHS must be part of it, from design to successful delivery.

More information on the NHS change model and guidance on how to use it can be found at www.nhsiq.nhs.uk.

IMPORTANCE OF MOTIVATION

An important aspect of generating any change is motivation. Why should we change? People are complex, and for any change to happen, it requires people to feel motivated enough to make it become a reality.

Frederick Herzberg (1968) studied what motivates us in the field of work and identified that there are some things we take for granted; however, if they are not there we become de-motivated and more negative. He called these hygiene factors. He also discovered that there are some things that, when present, positively motivate us. He called these motivator factors. Notice how contrary to what many people may believe, salary is not actually a motivator. However, if you take this away, it we will become a de-motivator (Table 4.3).

It is important to consider how you will motivate people when you are leading any change. What is it your followers believe in? What do they accept as givens and what will motivate them toward your future vision? A good leader will spend a lot of time on this before embarking on any change programme.

Have you considered what motivates you? Do the factors above resonate with you? What motivates your colleagues and stakeholders? By taking time out to consider and factor these into your work as a leader, you will more likely achieve positive results.

HOW WE REACT TO CHANGE

Stop and think about the last time a change was forced upon you that you weren't fully expecting. How did it make you feel? Research in the 1960s by Elisabeth Kubler-Ross (1969), which originated in how we deal with grief, demonstrated how generally human beings all respond similarly to change. Figure 4.6 explains the key stages that we go through.

Simply put, we can think of this in four key phases:

Phase 1 – Denial: After the initial shock, people will often deny the change is happening. They may avoid the topic, challenge the decision or refuse to believe it is happening.

Phase 2 – Resistance: People are likely to become angry, aggressive or at extremes become depressed and feel overwhelmed with the situation. *Note:* Some people will never go beyond this point in the curve without help. It is therefore the job of any good leader to help take their followers out of this negative place by providing support.

Phase 3 – Exploration: Here, people are more actively seeking to understand, accept or enhance the new ways of working. They may become creative and energised by the new world and seek ways to make the situation better.

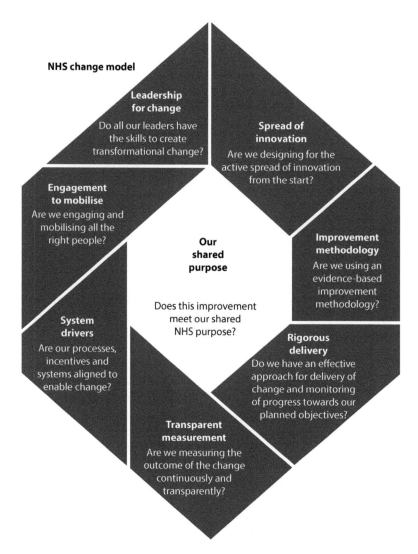

Figure 4.5 The NHS change model (NHS Improving Quality, 2013. http://www.nhsiq.nhs.uk/capacity-capability/nhs-change-model.aspx. With permission.)

Table 4.3 Motivator and hygiene factors

Motivator factors	Hygiene factors
Achievement	Company policy
Recognition	Supervision
Work itself	Relationship with boss
Responsibility	Work conditions
Promotion	Salary
Growth	Relationship with peers

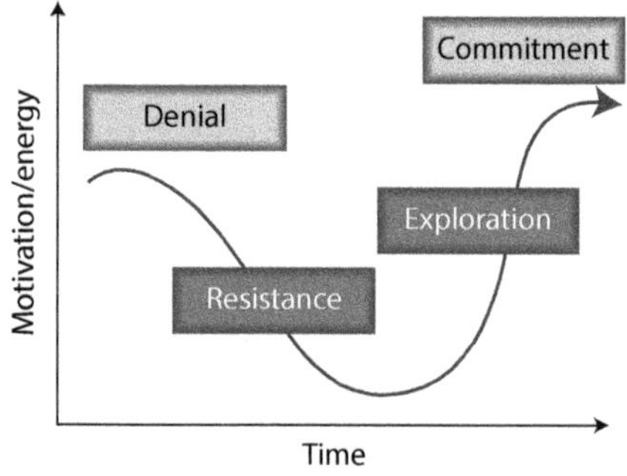

Figure 4.6 Kubler-Ross's (1969) stages of change.

Phase 4 – Commitment: People have accepted the change and are able to confidently resonate with the possibilities that it has brought. They then focus on continual improvement and work toward achieving results.

Can you reflect on a previous change that took place and recognise all of the stages you went through? How did you feel? What could you see? What were people around you doing and saying? Are you still mid-change and, if so, which point in the curve are you? And finally, what did you do to lead the way toward the positive future?

INFLUENCING PEOPLE

The ability to influence the actions and decisions of individuals and groups is a vital public health skill. An individual may be very skilled in analysing data or undertaking research, but if

EXERCISE 4.6: Assessing your change management skills

The following simple self-assessment has been adapted from work by Heller (1998). Use the tool (Table 4.4) to rate yourself against each of the questions to consider how well you are prepared to manage change:

Table 4.4 Change management skills self-assessment tool

	Question	Self-rating*
1	I am continuously thinking about what is impacting on my organisation and how I can positively respond to it	
2	I can think of times that I have helped make a challenging change into a success, or at least helped it significantly along the way	
3	I link what I am doing to the needs of my stakeholders, and ultimately the need of service users and patients within health and care	
4	I involve others in what I am trying to achieve	
5	I listen to people's views and perspectives, and will integrate them into my thinking, allowing me to adapt to an even better end vision	
6	I break down what I am trying to achieve into small bite-sized chunks	
7	I celebrate the successes of the work, both big and small, with those around me	
8	I recognise and reward people for their efforts when they support my work	
9	I seize opportunities when they present themselves	
10	I plan well ahead in order to ensure I am able to achieve my vision	
11	I learn from both mistakes and successes	
12	I develop those around me	
13	I often adapt and flex when obstacles challenge my work	
14	I pilot things and gather evidence to prove the need for change, before advising we should take a course of action	
15	I consider risks and plan for how to avoid, mitigate or overcome these	
16	I encourage others to support the vision and help them to lead with me	
17	I evaluate my work and learn from it	
18	I identify champions who will help me initiate my proposed change	

* Self-rating: 1 = never; 2 = sometimes; 3 = always

HOW DID YOU SCORE?

18–30: You are potentially new to change management. Don't worry! We all have to start somewhere. Do some wider learning around the topic and consider writing a reflective journal to help you understand what works and what doesn't within your workplace and professional role. This will help you gain confidence in leading change.

31–42: You likely understand the need for change and have probably helped support or lead a number of change initiatives. Keep embracing the opportunity to lead change projects and take time to evaluate what works, what doesn't and your preferred methods and tools for making change happen.

43–54: You are likely to be a skilled change agent who has led many change initiatives in the past. Think about what made the changes successful, what challenges you faced and what you did personally to make them into a success. Also, think about how you can help others achieve successful changes.

they have not developed their influencing skills, either in writing or in person, they may lose the opportunity to really make improvements or changes.

Establishing evidence, facts and viewpoints is crucial, but the method and skills used to present them are also vital.

There are many day-to-day examples where you have an opportunity to influence people; think about your day. Some may include:

- Writing a report or briefing for senior colleagues
- Making presentations to professionals
- Compiling and presenting data to a local government official
- Conversing with partners on the telephone
- Conducting large or small meetings with colleagues

EMOTIONAL INTELLIGENCE

According to the *Oxford Dictionary*, emotional intelligence can be defined as 'the capacity to be aware of, control, and express one's emotions, and to handle interpersonal relationships judiciously and empathetically'.

> IQ contributes about 20% to the factors that determine life success, which leaves 80% to other sources. (Goleman, 1995)

There are four types of emotional intelligence abilities as, adapted from Salovey and Mayer (1990)

- *Perceiving emotions:* Ability to identify emotions in faces and voices and the ability to detect your own emotions
- *Using emotions:* Ability to use emotions to support the process of problem solving or decision making
- *Understanding emotions:* Ability to understand what causes emotions, their progressions and interactions among emotions
- *Managing emotions:* Ability to regulate emotions in yourself and in others to enhance decision making and gain progress

For a case study on using emotional intelligence see Box 4.1.

EXERCISE 4.7

Consider the four types of emotional intelligence abilities described above and reflect on situations where you have used each of the types. These may be examples from home or work.

Reflect on the types of emotional intelligence during one-to-one and group situations. Do you work with someone with good emotional intelligence? What can you learn from them?

BOX 4.1: Case study

You meet with a local government official, Councillor Roodowse, who wants to know why air pollution is not a priority. Councillor Roodowse is sitting with arms crossed and tells you in a clipped voice that residents in their constituency are complaining of poor air quality and that asthma is rampant in the people who live there. You empathise with her frustrations and use information that you have to show Councillor Roodowse that air quality is a priority in certain areas; however, recent measurements of air quality in her constituency fall within reasonable limits and the asthma diagnoses are normal for the type of population living in her constituency. You ask questions about the views of constituents and find that residents are concerned with proposed housing developments in their area. You share knowledge, check understanding and offer to help draft a response to constituents.

Emotional intelligence type	Method
Perceiving emotions	You accurately identify that Councillor Roodowse feels frustrated by recognising facial expressions, body language and tone of voice.
Using emotions	You empathise with the frustrated emotion Councillor Roodowse is experiencing and you can relate through evidence in other areas.
Understanding emotions	You know you have to move Councillor Roodowse from a frustrated to an understanding and accepting emotion. You do not want Councillor Roodowse to become more frustrated.
Managing emotions	You acknowledge the frustration of Councillor Roodowse and her constituents and question how the feelings have arisen. You manage emotions by offering knowledge and offering to support the councillor in responding.

APPLICATION IN YOUR ROLE

Opportunities to influence people and groups arise in different work situations:

- Written approaches – from email through to formal board reports
- Telephone calls and visual media
- Meetings – both one-to-one meetings and group meetings
- Presentations
- Media – press releases, live or recorded radio and television segments

The audience you wish to influence will also vary (Table 4.5).

PREPARING FOR A MEETING

You may attend regular meetings in your role. Meetings provide an opportunity for you to communicate and influence others.

EXERCISE 4.8: Think about regular meetings you attend

- What makes a meeting successful – attendance, the chairperson, an agenda?
- Do you attend meetings that don't seem to achieve much? Why do you think this is?
- What do you do to prepare yourself for a meeting?

Table 4.5 Types of audiences that public health professionals interact with

Audience	Example
Public health and healthcare staff – clinical or management	• Briefing your director of public health, local primary healthcare leader or hospital chief executive in preparation for a committee or board meeting • Meeting with commissioning partners (e.g. NHS England, Public Health England, other local government authorities) • Meeting with a healthcare professional involved in providing a service (e.g. general practitioner (GP), midwife)
Local government and non-health service public health specialists or partners	• Meeting or a briefing with local government senior professions (e.g. director of children's services, director of social care or director of education) on a public health issue • Meeting with other senior officers or charity leads to discuss public health role or actions (e.g. local food bank, transport lead, occupational health, children's centres' lead, carers' charity)
Media and politicians	• Media interview or briefing, including mock telephone, radio, TV or print • Press officers of local organisations • Meeting with a local councillor
Members of the public and lay groups	• Meeting with members of the public on an issue specific to them or a family member • Meeting with a representative of a lobby group or residents' forum

Practising public health tip 4.2 Successful meetings: Use your language, approach and structure to convey what you can offer and what you need in a meeting:

- Identify who you will be meeting and frame your preparation around this information.
- Draw up a brief agenda or structure to guide your discussion.
- Sum up what you believe was agreed in the meeting at the end so everyone leaves with the same understanding of actions/decisions.

Preparing for a meeting should mean more than ensuring that you're in the right place at the right time with the right papers. Understanding who you're meeting or who your audience is beforehand will enable you to frame your viewpoints and arguments successfully. A good chair and an agenda will ensure that time is well used and that all contributions are considered.

UNDERSTANDING CURRENT PUBLIC HEALTH PRIORITIES AND POLICIES

Keeping up to date with current priorities and policies relevant to public health and the wider organisation you work in will enable you to see the bigger picture of your role and that of your team.

EXERCISE 4.9

Consider the key members of staff or teams you work with

- What are the key priorities and policies that influence their work?

If you're unsure, speak to each team to ask them for an overview or arrange a workshop where teams can share and reflect on the priorities and policies in their area.

There are several ways to identify new public health priority areas and policies:

- Sign up for bulletins from relevant organisations; examples in the UK are the King's Fund, gov.uk digest, the National Institute for Health and Care Excellence (NICE) and your local university.
- Read through previous agendas and minutes from local multidisciplinary health committees.

Practising public health tip 4.3 Providing context: To provide context for public health discussions, familiarise and refresh yourself with:

- Key **priority issues** (e.g. dementia, wider determinants of health, obesity, mental wellbeing)
- Key **overarching policy areas** in public health in the last 2–3 years (e.g. preventative care and reablement, community resilience, integration of health and social care services, sustainable models of funding)

You do not need to be an expert in each area and issue, but an overview will enable you to tackle situations with up-to-date knowledge and provide context to your discussions.

PROJECT MANAGEMENT

Project management is the process and activity of planning, organising, motivating and controlling resources (such as people or money), procedures and protocols to achieve specific goals (Table 4.6).

Table 4.6 Stages and tools of project management

Stage/area	Methods
Plan	• Action plan • Gantt chart • Stakeholder analysis • Communications and consultation and input from service users' SMART objectives – specific, measureable, attainable, relevant, time-bound
Implement	• Pilot study • PDSA cycles – plan, do, study, act • Regular team meetings • Stakeholder input
Review and improve	• Evaluation • Audit • Performance management

SUCCESSFUL PARTNERSHIP WORKING

Working in partnership can mean working with other organisations and services or with individuals and groups such as service users or patients. Partnership working involves establishing and developing inclusive, supportive and mutually beneficial relationships or wider working groups to improve the quality and delivery of services and functions. In many ways, the contemporary thinking we have already covered around systems leadership is highly important to enabling successful partnership working.

Effective partnership working should result in good quality services and functions with the respective roles and responsibilities of all parties identified and brought together under a structure.

EXERCISE 4.10

What partners do you currently work with in your area of work?

Are there any other partners that could be involved that would enhance your area of work?

Think:

- Communities, individuals and groups
- Statutory sector
- Voluntary sector
- Independent sector

Types of partnership

Table 4.7 outlines the ways that organisations interact.

Benefits of partnership working can include:

- Sharing of resources including finance, skills and information
- Improving efficiency through coordination, streamlining and rationalisation of processes and functions as each group fulfils their specific role
- Improving the planning and commissioning of services that complement rather than duplicate or disrupt each other
- Providing an opportunity to 'get it right the first time' by involving and including all relevant stakeholders meaningfully

Characteristics of bad partnerships can include:

- Lack of engagement by some members leading to conflict and a loss of trust
- No overall responsibility for partnership's delivery with no decision maker(s) identified
- Seen as a good thing to do, but not a priority for any partner (are different representatives sent to each meeting?)
- Meetings are used as a talking shop or breather from the day job

Barriers to partnership working and risks can include:

- Agencies and organisations facing different priorities, governmental direction and performance management arrangements
- Technical and infrastructure problems, including budget pressures, terms and conditions of staff, different IT systems and different governance arrangements

English policy and legislation on joint working include:

- Under Section 75 of the NHS Act (2006), NHS organisations and local authorities in England can pool budgets, join staff and management structures together and delegate commissioning responsibilities to each other.
- The Local Government and Public Involvement in Health Act (2007) requires local authorities to produce joint strategic needs assessments (JSNAs) of the health and wellbeing of their populations to shape joint planning of services.

How do you lead from within a partnership?

Leading from within and across partnerships is a challenge that public health professionals are increasingly facing head on. Public health is like a node interfacing with multiple agencies, trying to lead on improving health and wellbeing on behalf of our diverse population. And it's hard – how can you please everyone? Therefore what public health cannot do is achieve this alone. This is why working in partnership is so important.

Figure 4.7 illustrates contemporary research within healthcare that identifies cyclical stages that a partnership may go through and the leadership

Table 4.7 Different ways in which organisations and services work together

Type	Characteristics	Example
Cooperate	Partners may share information No joint planning; resources are kept separate	• Strategic partnerships – e.g. local safeguarding boards
Coordinate	Partners will do some planning together Sharing of responsibilities, resources and risks	• Multidisciplinary teams from different backgrounds • Pooled budgets
Collaborate	Organisational changes so that there is a higher degree of shared leadership, control, resources and risk sharing	• Structural integration of organisations and management teams • Joint commissioning of services

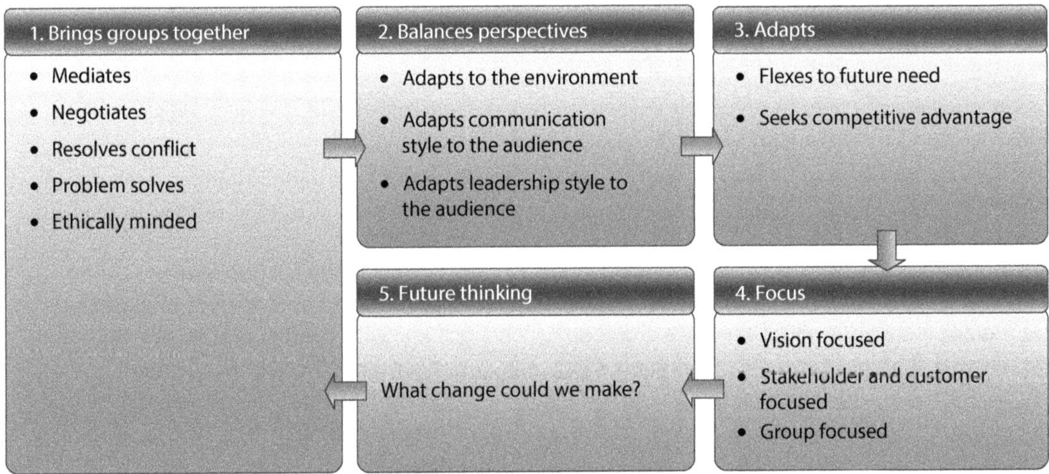

Figure 4.7 The five pillars of partner-leader skills and qualities. (From Turner A. 2012. *Health Service Journal*, July, 30–32. With permission.)

qualities that may be relevant to each stage. It may be useful to consider the stage that the partnerships you are working with are currently at, and the skills you may require to lead and facilitate effective partnership working in the future. Remember, it's a cycle and the partnership can spring between stages.

A further consideration is how do you structure and position the partnership to be fully effective and influential? It may help to think of the

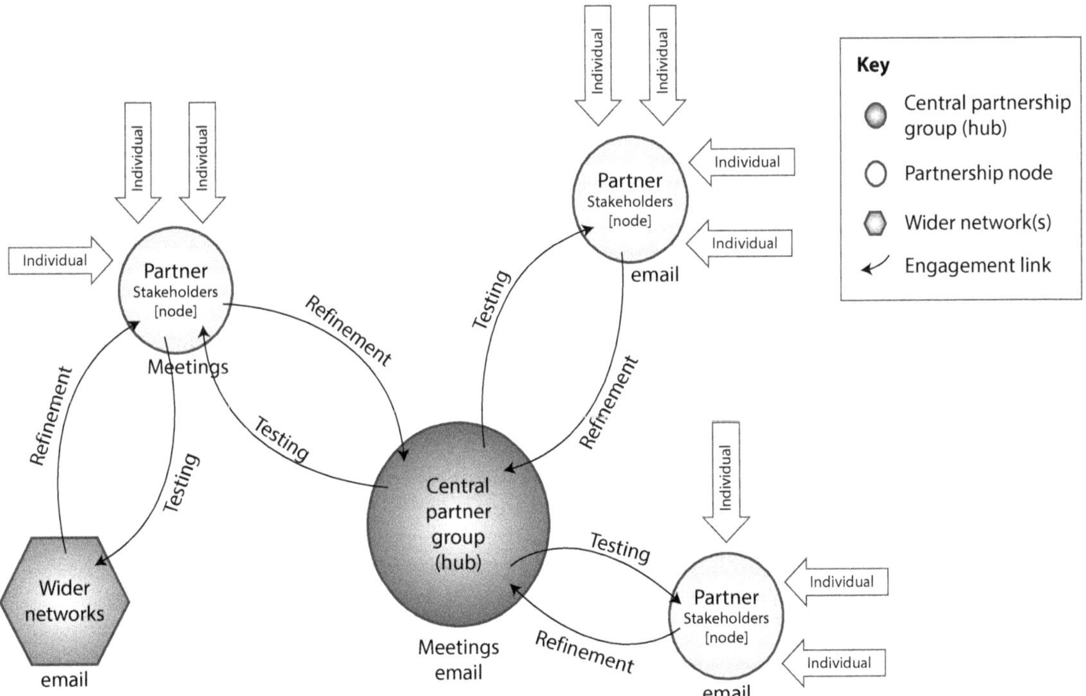

Figure 4.8 Example of a networking, engagement and collaborative working partnership model. (From Turner A. 2012. *Health Service Journal*, July, 30–32. With permission.)

EXERCISE 4.11: Is your partnership healthy?

Consider the lists of statements below in relation to a partnership you're involved with. Tick any statements that you feel apply.

Leadership
The partnership ...

- □ Shares a common vision
- □ Demonstrates added value
- □ Has members that are willing to make changes
- □ Has a leader that facilitates partnership working
- □ Has objectives of all partners aligned

Performance
The partnership ...

- □ Has a structure that fits its purpose
- □ Has clearly defined roles, responsibilities and contributions
- □ Has objectives, targets and milestones that are set and owned
- □ Has adequate resources
- □ Has project management and coordination

Trust
Members ...

- □ Are mutually accountable
- □ Understand and respect differences
- □ Deal with conflict and frustration
- □ Have effective communication
- □ Share contributions, risks and rewards
- □ Have equal say

Learning
Members ...

- □ Continuously seek improvements
- □ Review the partnership
- □ Seek to learn from each other
- □ Use strengths and talents

Look at the statements above that you have ticked and any gaps. Do the gaps lie mostly in any one area? What can you do to make improvements in your partnership?

- Identify strategic and operational leads from each partner.
- Clarify whether the agenda is a priority for each partner.
- Ask members what could be done differently.
- Ask leaders or the board to clarify if the subject is a priority.
- Identify leadership and accountability focus.

partnership sitting within a networked system. Your core partnership group is a central node, interfacing in many ways with other groups. You will send out and seek information through members, communications and wider mechanisms and receive information back to enable work to progress.

Figure 4.8 illustrates a model developed within healthcare to conceptualise this. Enabling the partnership to interface in such a networked way will extend its influence and what it can achieve. As part of this model, what is highly important is face-to-face contact. Effective partnerships are made up of real people and therefore require authentic partners to interface with them to help them to succeed.

FURTHER READING

For a more in-depth introduction to leadership: Northouse PG. 2004. *Leadership: Theory and Practice*. 3rd ed. London: Sage Publications.

5

Relevance to public health assessments and examinations

ADAM D M BRIGGS

Introduction 87
Part A Membership Examination of the FPH of the Royal Colleges of Physicians 87
Part B Membership Examination of the FPH of the Royal Colleges of Physicians: Objective Structured Public Health Examination 88
Exam structure and preparation 89
UK public health specialty training curriculum 91
UK Public Health Register 92
Public health skills and knowledge framework 92

INTRODUCTION

This book has been written to help public health professionals be as effective as possible in their day-to-day jobs.

It also will help with examinations and assessments that have a communication element. Although the details of formal competency requirements for different professional bodies are likely to change over time, the key skills that need to be demonstrated will likely stay the same. Therefore the detail of different assessments provided below may change slightly, and we would recommend checking the websites of the relevant professional bodies for the most up-to-date information.

This textbook has a particular focus on the Faculty of Public Health (FPH) of the Royal Colleges of Physicians (UK) Part B membership examination, the Objective Structured Public Health Examination (OSPHE), on which the scenarios in Chapter 6 are based, but can help with other public health professional assessments outlined below.

PART A MEMBERSHIP EXAMINATION OF THE FPH OF THE ROYAL COLLEGES OF PHYSICIANS

Written communication skills are tested in the Part A examination – candidates are expected to be capable of handling information and using the media in advising the public about health services, disease prevention (including communicable disease outbreaks and environmental hazards) and health promotion. Along with Mastering Public Health (Lewis et al., 2014), this book provides tips to help candidates successfully answer relevant questions in the Part A exam, and to demonstrate a practical understanding of the issues discussed.

PART B MEMBERSHIP EXAMINATION OF THE FPH OF THE ROYAL COLLEGES OF PHYSICIANS: OBJECTIVE STRUCTURED PUBLIC HEALTH EXAMINATION

Verbal and listening communication skills are the key element in this examination, and this book provides comprehensive coverage of the abilities that need to be demonstrated in order to pass the OSPHE. The practising public health tips interspersed throughout the book are particularly relevant to the examination.

The FPH website describes the OSPHE as a 'show how' assessment of the candidate's ability to apply relevant knowledge, skills and attitudes to the practice of public health. The training section of the FPH website contains details of the OSPHE's content (http://www.fph.org.uk).

Along with the Part A examination, the OSPHE is required for nomination as a member of the FPH and is a prerequisite for those in the public health specialty training programme to gain their certificate of completion of training.

In the OSPHE, candidates are assessed against five main competencies and across four topic areas; the same five competencies being repeatedly and independently tested in each of six scenarios (Davison et al., 2010). Box 5.1 outlines these competencies and topic areas, as reported by the FPH.

The chapters of this book have used a range of examples that are illustrative of the types of scenarios that a candidate may expect to encounter in the OSPHE. Box 5.2 shows the four types of scenarios, including examples, published on the FPH website.

BOX 5.1: Competencies and topic areas assessed by the MFPH Part B OSPHE examination*

COMPETENCIES ASSESSED

1. The ability to demonstrate **presenting communication skills** (verbal and non-verbal) appropriately in typical public health settings: presenting to a person or audience
2. The ability to demonstrate **listening and comprehending communication skills** (verbal and non-verbal) appropriately in typical public health settings: listening and responding appropriately
3. The ability to assimilate **relevant information** from a variety of sources and settings and using it appropriately from a public health perspective
4. The ability to demonstrate **appropriate reasoning, analytical and judgement skills**, giving a balanced view within public health settings
5. The ability to handle uncertainty, the unexpected, challenge and conflict appropriately

TOPIC AREAS FROM WHICH SCENARIOS WILL BE DRAWN

1. **Health protection** (including infection, immunisation, screening and environmental subject matter).
2. **Health promotion and health improvement** (including lifestyle and behavioural interventions at individual and population levels, partnership working and wider determinants of health).
3. **Quality healthcare: Technical aspects** of commissioning which require expert advice or assessment utilising public health skills. Examples include the application of technical material to health or healthcare provision.
4. **Quality healthcare: Implementation** of health or healthcare interventions and working with patients, the public, professionals or organisations.

* From the training section of the FPH website http://www.fph.org.uk/.

BOX 5.2: Scenario types that may be encountered in the OSPHE*

1. **Media/high-profile 'public'**: Media – newspaper, radio pre-recorded; member of Parliament or local council leader; press officer of the National Health Service (NHS) or partner organisation
2. **Other non-health service public health 'specialist'/key 'public health improvement' partner**: Meeting with/briefing for senior professional (e.g. professional whose job focus has strong public health element such as director of children's services or an informed chair of a non-health or other organisation); meeting with or briefing for new public health (PH) trainees or non-specialist staff; meeting with other senior officer of council or other partner organisation to discuss PH actions
3. **The lay public**: Meeting with local councillor/non-NHS health partnership chair or member; meeting with member of the public on an issue pertinent to them; meeting with representative of patient forum or pressure or lobby group
4. **Healthcare staff – clinical and general management**: Briefing to chair of NHS committee or board (non-clinical); meeting with healthcare manager – commissioner or chief executive or other senior; meeting with healthcare professional involved in care delivery – general practitioner (GP)/consultant/nurse/Allied health professional.

* From the training section of the FPH website http://www.fph.org.uk/.

EXAM STRUCTURE AND PREPARATION

This book outlines all the practical public health skills required for the OSPHE. Practising scenarios with colleagues and supervisors under examination conditions is essential to ensure that you are aware of the exam's format, the layout of presented materials and the time constraints. Although the exam material is carefully edited to make sure there are no English, Scottish, Welsh or Northern Irish specific scenarios, the material does broadly refer to UK examples and as such is focused on the practice of public health within a Westernised state-funded healthcare system.

The exam is 1 hour 48 minutes long and consists of six stations, each lasting eight minutes. Before each station, candidates will be given some key written information relating to the station's content and the objectives of the scenario. There is then eight minutes to prepare for the station in a room on your own before moving into a room with the examiner and the actor to begin the scenario. One minute is allowed for the transfer between rooms. Of note, the FPH can pilot new scenarios during examinations, and the results of these stations will not count toward your final score. There is up-to-date detailed information on what to expect on the day available in the examination section of the FPH website, and for any questions, it is best to contact the relevant FPH officers (http://www.fph.org.uk/).

The FPH website has a range of scenarios available for practice. Each includes content for the candidate, examiner and actor, and instructions for running the scenario. Extra FPH scenarios (not available on the FPH website) are reproduced in Chapter 6. Candidates often find it difficult to understand how well they have done in this exam and so in Chapter 6 we put the reader in the role of the examiner so you can benchmark how you think eight candidates scored against the FPH competencies listed in Box 5.1. This, alongside feedback from FPH examiners, will help to illustrate the expected standard. The scenarios used in the OSPHE are mostly based on real-life situations that the scenario authors have encountered in the everyday practice of public health.

For tips from previously successful OSPHE candidates on the exam, see Box 5.3.

BOX 5.3: OSPHE tips

FPH examiners and successful public health specialty registrars have suggested some *do's* and *don'ts* that may help you both when preparing for the exam and on the day itself.

PREPARATION

- **Do's**

Do use a range of colleagues and friends to practise with (including people you don't know too well) – you could try using video conferencing to practise with candidates in other parts of the country (and turning off the video for the telephone-only stations).

Do go through your Part A notes as part of your preparation – these can be really useful for going over definitions of various concepts and providing frameworks for answering questions.

Do try and video yourself when practising. Watching them back might be awkward, but it can also help identify unhelpful body language and mannerisms that you may not have been aware of.

Do try and focus your preparation on your weaknesses. Do you need more practice on how best to use the 8 minutes preparation? Do you need to get more comfortable with how to open a conversation?

Do attend a practice OSPHE, either organised by your training programme or a formal course elsewhere in the country. These are a particularly useful way of experiencing the time pressures and having to move on between stations.

Do be wary of advice from commercial or other preparation exam courses around how to address each scenario with a prepared introduction or response. These can detract from your natural communication skills, hinder you really listening to what you are being asked, and are no substitute for knowing the subject and common sense communication skills.

Do think about using frameworks to help plan answers to common scenarios, such as dealing with an outbreak or developing a strategy.

Do have a think about a generic framework for approaching a scenario if you get stuck. For example: introduction (self), set the scene (background, importance of issue, and clarify the aims of the scenario), discussion, summarise, and close with agreed actions.

- **Don'ts**

Don't shy away from presenting in meetings when at work – the pressure and subsequent questions can be really useful experience for going into the Part B exam.

Don't prepare in isolation. Even if you don't want to practise with other people, candidates who have previously sat the exam will often have practice scenarios from courses or online resources that they can share.

Don't shy away from asking for and offering constructive criticism to colleagues both when practising scenarios and when at work.

Don't do all the practice scenarios early in your preparation so you have none left to look at in the week before the exam.

Don't spend too much time in the build-up to the exam solely working on public health analytical duties or report writing duties. Instead it is important to volunteer to do as many activities as possible that involve verbal interactions – instead optimise your 'front-line' public health duties.

EXAM DAY

- **Do's**

Do try to identify up to three key messages when preparing each station.

Do read the brief and answer the question – it's easy in the pressure of the exam to answer the question you want to answer rather than the one that's being asked.

Do simply introduce yourself beforehand. There's no need to waste time with a fabricated story about your department, and thank the actor and assessor afterwards.

Do keep it simple – overcomplicating things can lead to confusion, so focus on your key messages and avoid jargon.

Do draw diagrams or share the data in the pack with the actor if you think it may be helpful.

Do try and treat each station like a real situation as though you were at work – therefore try not to come out of character if you make a mistake.

Do be confident; try and maintain eye contact and open body language.

Do check understanding toward the end of each station and ask if the scenario actor has any questions.

Do try and finish with a summary, signpost to further resources, and make a follow-up plan.

Do be aware that sometimes the FPH chooses to record a station for training purposes and try not to be put off by this.

Do smile and try to enjoy it!

- **Don'ts**

Don't lie. Be honest when you don't know something. You are always able to say you'll get in touch again at another time with the answers to specific questions.

Don't respond to conflict by being confrontational. Try to acknowledge the problem, explain the situation and identify a possible plan or solution.

Don't linger on the previous station – try to forget how it went and focus on the next one with a clean slate.

Don't say more than you need to. Be succinct and the examiner will ask if they want more information.

Don't avoid uncertainty in either a question or data. Be explicit about it and say how you would deal with it.

Don't avoid non-scientific terms when they are for a specific part of the scenario; for example, don't use 'value for money' when you are being asked about cost-effectiveness, but instead explain what cost-effectiveness means in lay terms.

Don't be put off by the clocks – they can be quite loud!

UK PUBLIC HEALTH SPECIALTY TRAINING CURRICULUM

Public health specialty training in the UK is the General Medical Council (GMC) and UK FPH approved programme for individuals to become consultants in public health. As mentioned above, the MFPH examinations are a requirement for completion of training; however, these form just one part of the wider curriculum requirements (the full curriculum can be found under the training section of the FPH website, www.fph.org.uk, or through the education section of the GMC website, www.gmc-uk.org). The competencies assessed fall under nine key areas (Box 5.4).

Each key area has competencies requiring the demonstration of skills outlined in this book, ranging from delivering presentations to influencing

BOX 5.4: Competency key areas for UK public health specialty training

- **Key Area 1**: Surveillance and assessment of the population's heath and wellbeing
- **Key Area 2**: Assessing the evidence of effectiveness of health and healthcare interventions, programmes and services
- **Key Area 3**: Policy and strategy development and implementation
- **Key Area 4**: Strategic leadership and collaborative working for health
- **Key Area 5**: Health improvement
- **Key Area 6**: Health protection
- **Key Area 7**: Health and social service quality
- **Key Area 8**: Public health intelligence
- **Key Area 9**: Academic public health

people or dealing with conflict. More information on how to apply to be on the specialty registrar training programme can be found on the training pages of the FPH website (www.fph.org.uk).

UK PUBLIC HEALTH REGISTER

This book will assist with the skills required by public health professionals working toward membership of the UK Public Health Register (UKPHR). The standards required are framed around four areas of practice, each with a range of expected competencies:

1. Professional and ethical practice – this should be at the heart of everything a public health practitioner does.
2. Technical competencies in public health – these cover the essential knowledge and skills that anyone working in public health needs to have.
3. Application of public health competencies to public health work – this relates to the specific functions that public health practitioners undertake.
4. Underpinning skills and knowledge – this is needed by all public health practitioners to act effectively and achieve improvements in population health and wellbeing.

Communication skills will feed mainly into Areas 3 and 4 outlined above and will be of particular relevance to Competencies 9, 11 and 12 as outlined below.

Area 3: Application of technical competencies to public health work in particular:

Competency 9: Work collaboratively to plan and deliver programmes to improve health and wellbeing outcomes for populations/communities/groups/families/individuals – demonstrating:

9e. Awareness of the effect the media has on public perception
9f. How the health concerns and interests of individuals, groups and communities have been communicated
9g. How the prevention, amelioration or control of risks has been communicated

Area 4: Underpinning skills and knowledge in particular:

Competency 11: Work collaboratively with people from teams and agencies other than one's own to improve health and wellbeing outcomes – demonstrating:

11a. Awareness of personal impact on others
11b. Constructive relationships with a range of people who contribute to population health and wellbeing
11c. Awareness of:
    i. Principles of effective partnership working
    ii. The ways in which organisations, teams and individuals work together to improve health and wellbeing outcomes

Competency 12: Communicate effectively with a range of different people using different methods.

Details of how to join the UKPHR and the range of competencies required can be found on the UKPHR website, www.ukphr.org.

PUBLIC HEALTH SKILLS AND KNOWLEDGE FRAMEWORK

This framework outlines the comprehensive skills and knowledge needed across three groups of the workforce for public health: specialists (Levels 8–9), practitioners (Levels 5–7) and the wider public health workforce (Levels 1–4). It has been developed by Public Health Online Resource for Careers, Skills, and Training and is available on their website, www.phorcast.org.uk. The framework provides professionals and employers with the expected level of practice of public health professionals and allows public health professionals to identify gaps in their skill set as well as opportunities for professional development. This textbook will help provide knowledge and skills in some key areas.

The Public Health Skills and Knowledge Framework (PHSKF) is divided into nine areas. For each area there are details of the skills needed at each of the nine levels outlined above. Communication skills run through all the areas of the PHSKF and across all of the levels. The most relevant to the skills covered in this book are detailed below.

Surveillance and assessment of the population's health and wellbeing

Level 5: Communicate and disseminate findings on the health and wellbeing of a population to others.
Level 6: Present, communicate and disseminate data about health and wellbeing in a variety of ways as appropriate to different audiences.

Assessing the evidence of effectiveness of interventions, programmes and services to improve population health and wellbeing

Level 4: Communicate evidence to a defined audience.
Level 5: Communicate evidence to others.
Level 6: Communicate findings of the appraisal of evidence on a specific issue.
Level 9: Communicate and disseminate critically appraised evidence to key decision makers in different organisations.

Leadership and collaborative working to improve population health and wellbeing

Level 1: Communicate effectively with the people you work with.
Level 2: Communicate effectively with people related to your own work role to improve the population's health and wellbeing.
Level 3: Communicate with a range of people related to your own work role.
Level 4: Communicate for a range of purposes and with various audiences.
Level 5: Communicate using different techniques appropriate to the audience and the purpose of the communication.

Health improvement

Level 3: Communicate with people about their health and wellbeing and the actions they may take to achieve improvement.
Level 4: Communicate with individuals, groups and communities using various methods to enable them to improve health and wellbeing.
Level 4: Communicate to relevant people the health concerns and interests of individuals and communities.

Health protection

Level 3: Explain to individuals the reasons for monitoring risks and undertaking activities to protect health, wellbeing and safety.
Level 4: Communicate to individuals the risks to health, wellbeing and safety and advise how the risks can be prevented, ameliorated or controlled.
Level 5: Communicate risks to health, wellbeing and safety and provide advice to individuals on how to prevent, ameliorate or control the risks.
Level 6: Communicate risks to health, wellbeing and safety to individuals and communities and provide advice on how to prevent, ameliorate or control the risks.
Level 7: Prepare material for, and effectively use the media for, the communication of health messages.
Level 8: Manage risk communication on issues that are considered or perceived to be major threats to population health and wellbeing.
Level 9: Lead complex risk communication (particularly with the public) on issues that are considered or perceived to be major threats to population health, wellbeing and safety.

Public health intelligence

Level 8: Communicate and disseminate health data and intelligence from a wide range of sources to different populations.

Academic public health

Level 4: Disseminate research findings within area of work using methods appropriate to the audience.
Level 5: Disseminate research findings within area of work using methods that are appropriate to the audience.
Level 6: Communicate primary or secondary research findings using methods appropriate to the audience.
Level 8: Communicate complex issues that can affect health and wellbeing to a variety of audiences.

Health and social care quality

Level 3: Communicate appropriately with users of services.
Level 5: Communicate and disseminate information that improves practices/services.
Level 9: Engage with, and advise, strategic partners and decision makers to determine goals, priorities, targets, strategies, success criteria and outcome measures to achieve improvements in quality and patient/client/user safety.

6

Video scenarios

PAUL A FISHER, ROB F COOPER, JILL MEARA AND CHRIS PACKHAM

Introduction 95
Resources in this chapter 100
Scenario 1: Infection hazards of human cadavers 101
Scenario 2: Land contamination in a residential area 110
Scenario 3: Human papilloma virus (HPV) vaccine to prevent cervical cancer 117
Scenario 4: Interview on speed cameras 124
Scenario 5: Exceptional funding request 132
Scenario 6: Breast screening uptake rates 139
Scenario 7: Emergency hospital admissions 146
Scenario 8: Smoking ban 152
Part B scenario feedback forms completed by a team of experienced markers 158

INTRODUCTION

One of the best ways of demonstrating the practice of public health, including the skills of public health communication, is through observation. Therefore linked to this book are eight short videos of public health scenarios that can be accessed at the website provided for each one.

These scenarios are based on the Faculty of Public Health of the Royal Colleges of Physicians Part B: Objective Structured Public Health Examination (OSPHE). This exam aims to test competency in the practice of public health. Details can be found under the training section of its website (http://www.fph.org.uk) and in Box 6.1.

These videos represent a learning resource for all public health practitioners, not just those undertaking the Part B exam, as this exam is designed as a 'show how' assessment of the candidate's ability to apply relevant knowledge, skills and attitudes to the practice of public health.

The topics which cover the three domains of public health in a variety of common settings covered in the eight videos are detailed in Table 6.1.

To get the most out of the videos we suggest that you put yourself in the position of a candidate in the exam (i.e. read the candidate pack in eight minutes), watch a video and then put yourself in the position of an examiner (i.e. read the examiners pack and fill out a feedback sheet). Finally compare what you wrote in the feedback to what experienced examiners commented on in the completed forms at the end of the chapter (these steps are detailed in Box 6.2). Considering how you would have reacted in these situations will provide useful reflective learning opportunities to improve your practical public health skills.

BOX 6.1: Faculty of Public Health of the Royal Colleges of Physicians Part B: Objective Structured Public Health Examination (OSPHE)*

An individual taking the examination is assessed on five competences independently on six separate occasions. The competencies are

1. The ability to demonstrate **presenting communication skills** (verbal and non-verbal) appropriately in typical public health settings: presenting to a person or audience
2. The ability to demonstrate **listening and comprehending communication skills** (verbal and non-verbal) appropriately in typical public health settings: listening and responding appropriately
3. The ability to assimilate **relevant information** from a variety of sources and settings and using it appropriately from a public health perspective
4. The ability to demonstrate **appropriate reasoning, analytical and judgement skills**, giving a balanced view within public health settings
5. The ability to handle uncertainty, the unexpected, challenge and conflict appropriately

Marking guidance (for detailed guidance see Table 6.2) is given to marking examiners as to what to look out for in order to award one of the following grades:

A. **Excellent performance** – little room for improvement
B. **Good performance** – well above a satisfactory standard with some aspects which could be improved
C. **Satisfactory performance** – just above minimum acceptable standard
D. **Unsatisfactory but borderline** – some aspects acceptable but overall improvement needed in order to be acceptable public health practice
E. **Poor performance**

There is inevitably a degree of subjective judgement as to which mark to give – especially if a candidate is at the boundary between two grades. However, the same competencies repeatedly and independently tested six times make the overall assessment objective (and therefore a reliable measure of competency) (Davison et al., 2010).

* See examination section of the FPH website: http://www.fph.org.uk/

Table 6.1 Topics and participants in the eight videos

Scenario 1	**Infection Hazards of Human Cadavers** Role player: Mamoona Tahir, Consultant in Communicable Disease Control, PHE Public Health (candidate): Clare Walker, Specialty Registrar in Public Health
Scenario 2	**Land Contamination in a Residential Area** Role player: Paul Fisher, Specialty Registrar in Public Health Public Health (candidate): Ansaf Azhar, Specialty Registrar in Public Health
Scenario 3	**HPV Vaccine to Prevent Cervical Cancer** Role player: Dan Todkill, Specialty Registrar in Public Health Public Health (candidate): Adam Briggs, Specialty Registrar in Public Health
Scenario 4	**Interview on Speed Cameras** Role player: Nigel Smith, Health and Wellbeing, PHE Public Health (candidate): Dan Todkill, Specialty Registrar in Public Health
Scenario 5	**Exceptional Funding Request** Role player: Sally Bradshaw, Specialty Registrar in Public Health Public Health (candidate): Clare Walker, Specialty Registrar in Public Health
Scenario 6	**Breast Screening Uptake Rates** Role player: Carol Chatt, Specialty Registrar in Public Health Public Health (candidate): Sally Bradshaw, Specialty Registrar in Public Health
Scenario 7	**Emergency Hospital Admissions** Role player: Adam Briggs, Specialty Registrar in Public Health Public Health (candidate): Carol Chatt, Specialty Registrar in Public Health
Scenario 8	**Smoking Ban** Role player: Nigel Smith, Health and Wellbeing, PHE Public Health (candidate): Paul Fisher, Specialty Registrar in Public Health

Note: The registrars involved were acting and their performance in no way reflects their actual competencies (all have passed the Part B OSPHE exam). They are all thanked for performing, at times, intentionally and uncharacteristically poorly to enable common weaknesses to be highlighted in these videos.

BOX 6.2: How to use the videos

The best way to use these videos is to prepare as if taking the exam. Therefore:

- Step 1 – read the candidate pack for the scenario (these can be found later in this chapter).
- Step 2 – take 8 minutes to think how you would approach the situation.
- Step 3 – watch the video (the web address for each scenario can be found at the top of the relevant feedback form).
- Step 4 – note the good and bad communication tactics that were utilised and how the other competencies are demonstrated or otherwise.
- Step 5 – read the main marker examiner pack with a particular focus on the marking guide for examiners to see what the examiners are looking for.
- Step 6 – mark the candidate A (excellent), B (good), C (satisfactory), D (not satisfactory) or E (poor) for each of the five competencies below (there are eight blank feedback forms to use for steps 4 and 5); definitions for the A–E marking scheme are given in Table 6.2.
- Step 7 – compare your comments and marks with the completed feedback forms at the end of this chapter.

There is no need to watch these videos in any particular order as they are all stand-alone exercises.

Table 6.2 General marking criteria for the Part B MFPH

Competency	Grade	Criteria
1. The ability to demonstrate presenting communication skills (verbal and non-verbal) appropriately in typical public health settings	A	As B, plus demonstrates superior presentation skills: concise, articulate and persuasive. Conveys confidence and appropriate demeanour for scenario. Clearly engages with audience.
	B	As C, plus above-average presentation skills. Demonstrates confidence and understanding of the nature of the audience.
	C	Avoids jargon. Is clear. Appropriate language for the audience. Maintains eye contact. Appropriate manner for the scenario. Demonstrates empathy and politeness.
	D	Gross failure of one criterion of C or minor failure of two. Presents clearly but fails to show empathy or demonstrate an appropriate manner for the scenario or shows empathy and appropriate manner but presentation is muddled and not clear.
	E	Gross failure of more than one criterion of C or minor failure of more than two. Inarticulate. Tends toward impolite or patronising. Failure to understand nature of audience.
2. The ability to demonstrate listening and comprehending skills (verbal and non-verbal) appropriately in typical public health settings	A	As B, plus demonstrates complete understanding of questions and the situation. Anticipates further questions.
	B	As C, plus answers totality of questions. Demonstrates understanding of concerns.
	C	Listens and responds appropriately – manner of responses appropriate to scenario.
	D	Gross failure of one criterion of C or minor failure of two. Shows understanding but does not directly or appropriately answer questions. Demonstrates distraction or irritation at questions or lack of understanding for concerns.
	E	Gross failure of more than one criterion of C. Failure to understand questions and respond appropriately. Inability to follow discussion.
3. The ability to assimilate relevant information from a variety of sources and settings and using it appropriately from a public health perspective	A	As B, plus evidence of extensive background knowledge. Demonstrates superior public health skills relevant to the scenario.
	B	As C, plus evidence of additional and appropriate knowledge. Demonstrates additional practical public health skills relevant to the scenario and additional analysis of the information presented.

(Continued)

Table 6.2 (*Continued*) General marking criteria for the Part B MFPH

Competency	Grade	Criteria
	C	Shows sound knowledge by assimilating the key public health facts from the data provided. Satisfactorily explains the appropriate key public health concepts. Applies relevant knowledge to the scenario.
	D	Gross failure of one criterion of C or minor failure of two. Shows some but not all of the relevant knowledge and partial application of that knowledge. One error as defined by specific marking guidance. Candidate also demonstrates some lack of understanding of the data presented.
	E	Gross failure of more than one criterion of C or minor failure of more than two. Serious misinterpretation of the data presented. Makes serious errors as defined by the specific marking guidance. No demonstration of the proper application of public health principles.
4. The ability to demonstrate appropriate reasoning, analytical and judgement skills, giving a balanced view within public health settings	A	As B, plus demonstrates superior analytical and judgement skills relevant to the scenario. Provides innovative and local examples relevant to the scenario demonstrating superior application skills.
	B	As C, plus demonstrates additional practical public health skills relevant to the scenario and added insight based on a combination of knowledge, experience and the data presented.
	C	Demonstrates appropriate reasoning, analytical and judgement skills. Satisfactorily interprets and balances evidence. Provides clear explanations of appropriate key public health concepts. Applies relevant knowledge to the scenario.
	D	Gross failure of one criterion of C or minor failure of two. Shows some but not all of the relevant knowledge and partial application of that knowledge. Unclear explanations. Demonstrates bias or limited reasoning, analytical or judgement skills. One error as defined by specific marking guidance.
	E	Gross failure of more than one criterion of C or minor failure of more than two. Serious errors in explanations or no explanations or lack of understanding. Demonstrates poor/no reasoning, analytical or judgement skills. No balance in the interpretation of evidence. Makes serious errors as defined by the specific marking guidance.

(*Continued*)

Table 6.2 (*Continued*) General marking criteria for the Part B MFPH

Competency	Grade	Criteria
5. The ability to handle uncertainty, the unexpected, challenge and conflict appropriately	A	As B, plus demonstrates confidence and empathy in responding to challenging questions. Successfully addresses or anticipates concerns that are raised.
	B	As C, plus demonstrates sound appreciation of the concerns and difficulties involved.
	C	Responds to confrontation and challenging questions in a sensitive manner appropriate to the situation. Non-confrontational. Acknowledges uncertainty. Demonstrates a balanced style.
	D	Gross failure of one criterion of C or minor failure of two. Demonstrates uncertainty when challenged. Fails to fully appreciate the concerns and difficulties presented by the scenario.
	E	Gross failure of more than one criterion of C or minor failure of more than two. Candidate displays uncertainty and lack of clarity in responding to questions. Confrontational or patronising. Fails to address concerns raised. Muddled and self-contradictory responses.

Note: The Faculty of Public Health works hard to ensure consistency in the format of the questions at each sitting. The following eight scenarios are taken from sittings across several years and do not have the same level of consistency that a candidate would meet in a current exam sitting.

A, excellent; B, good; C, satisfactory; D, not satisfactory; E, poor.

RESOURCES IN THIS CHAPTER

The remainder of this chapter consists of:

- Eight blank feedback forms
- Eight scenarios – each one has a candidate pack (for the person taking the exam), a marker pack (for the person grading the exam) and a role player briefing pack (for the person playing the role of the individual the examinee is speaking to)
- Eight scenario feedback forms completed with comments and scores by experienced Part B examiners

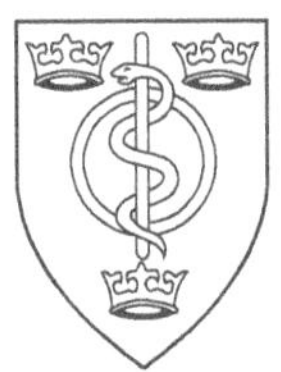

Faculty of Public Health

Of the Royal Colleges of Physicians of the United Kingdom

Working to improve the public's health

Scenario 1

Infection hazards of human cadavers

(original author Daniel Seddon, edited by Chris Packham and Jill Meara)

Candidate pack

CANDIDATE TASK

You are a trainee in a health protection unit.* You have recently completed a training assignment on environmental health issues within the construction industry. You have been asked to meet the union representative of workers on a local construction site. They wish to talk about concerns about possible health hazards from clearing a nineteenth-century burial site and the precautions that the workers need to take.

You have 8 minutes to prepare for the station. You are not required to prepare any visual aids. You will then spend 8 minutes discussing the task with a role player. You may use paper notes to aid your verbal briefing.

OUTLINE OF SITUATION

There is a major construction project to build a big shopping and entertainment complex in the local large town. The site for the new complex includes an old burial ground, which was in use throughout the nineteenth century and the early part of the twentieth century. The burial ground needs to be excavated and all the human remains removed.

The senior trade union official for the construction workers at the site has asked for a meeting to discuss the possible hazards associated with clearing burial sites. They have already sought advice from a national health and safety regulator. Neither they nor their members feel confident that the national health and safety regulator† is competent to advise on health issues such as this, and so now they wish to get further assurance from the local public health (health protection) specialists.

CANDIDATE GUIDANCE

Read the outline and briefing material and be prepared to answer the union representative's questions. He or she is concerned about the health risks of working with old interments (burials) and the appropriate precautions.

AT THE STATION

You will be greeted by a marker examiner who will take your candidate number and name and then hand over to the role player by saying:

> This is the trade union representative for the construction team. They will now start the station.

CANDIDATE BRIEFING PACK

Edited extracts from Healing TD, Hoffman PN, and Young SEJ, The infection hazards of human cadavers, *Communicable Disease Report* 5: R61–R68, 1995.

TYPES OF OLD INTERMENTS

By the 1840s, space in burial grounds in many towns in the UK was very limited. Coffins were

* Health protection unit is the local branch of a national body that provides specialists responsible for community infectious and non-infectious hazard control.

† The national health and safety regulator has the statutory duty to ensure companies abide by the relevant safety at work legislation. They have an enforcement and an advisory arm.

often stacked several deep in churchyards, with little earth cover. Burial grounds had to be cleared out frequently and remains re-interred in charnel pits (see below). Building work in the older parts of towns in Britain is quite likely to uncover human remains. Occasionally, large collections of human bones are discovered, which may be the remains of an overcrowded churchyard, plague pit or charnel pit.

Bones found in charnel pits can be arranged randomly or may be arranged as, for example, collections of skulls or long bones. Charnel pits are not hazardous because the disarticulated bones they contain have already been exposed to decay.

When epidemics occurred, whether in town or country, it was often impossible to bury all the dead in individual graves and the authorities tended to resort to mass burials (plague pits). The locations of larger pits are often indicated in parish records, but small unrecorded pits are sometimes found. In plague pits the remains tend to be found in the form of the human skeleton unless they have been disturbed by previous building activities or land movements. Plague pits present no hazards, because bodies were usually interred without coffins. The organisms that caused disease leading to mass death in the past do not survive well outside living hosts and are unlikely to withstand the intense microbial competition that occurs in decay. Many of those interred in graves in previous centuries may have died from infectious diseases such as plague, cholera, typhoid and tuberculosis. The organisms that cause these four diseases are unlikely to survive long in a buried cadaver, even in mass burials such as plague pits, and do not present a hazard.

PATHOGENS THAT MAY BE ASSOCIATED WITH OLD BURIALS

The risks posed by anthrax and smallpox are less clear, but are very low indeed.

Although anthrax is a potential risk because it can form highly resistant spores, large numbers of spores are very unlikely to be found in bodies in old burial sites. The risk is low because:

- Although the spores can last for long periods in dry conditions, spore formation occurs only under aerobic conditions and extensive spores could only be formed in association with a human cadaver if blood containing the organism had been spilt at the time of death.
- Anthrax has been an uncommon cause of death in Britain for 200 years, so infected corpses are most unlikely to be found.
- Humans are moderately resistant to anthrax and unlikely to be infected even if in contact with an infected cadaver.

Britain has been largely free of smallpox since 1935 (a few sporadic cases occurred after this date). The risk that smallpox might re-emerge if the remains of smallpox victims are disturbed appears to be remote. The virus is thought unlikely to survive in scabs in interments for more than a year. Morphologically intact orthopox virus was seen by electron microscopy of tissue from bodies more than 100 years old found in a crypt in Spitalfields, East London in 1985, but the virus could not be grown and was not thought to be infective.

PRECAUTIONS

Regardless of the age of a burial, residual soft tissue is a potential hazard, and if present, expert medical advice should be obtained from a local specialist in infection control. This is particularly important with well-preserved or mummified bodies, and even more so if skin lesions are seen.

In many instances when old interments are disturbed, the dead are found in coffins. Old coffins in good condition should be removed intact and reburied, but they are often fragile and should be sleeved in very heavy-duty sealed plastic before being moved. Wooden coffins have been used for many centuries, but lead coffins with or without wooden covers or linings can also be found.

Any inhalation hazards associated with disturbing old interments are likely to be greater in crypts and other enclosed spaces than in the open air. Pathogens associated with cadavers are likely to pose less risk than lead dust and coffin wood, which may be contaminated with mould or parasite eggs, or powdered by wood-boring insects. Protection against these hazards will also protect against any remote risk of infection. Protective equipment should include overalls, head coverings, safety helmets, gloves, face shields and high-quality dust masks.

Chloride of lime (quicklime) should not be used as a disinfectant during exhumations. It is not particularly effective and is hazardous to the workforce.

Burial ground clearance has not been that uncommon over the last half century, but transmission of 'dread disease' from cadavers to those clearing the burial site has not been documented.

Examiner pack

EXAMINER SITUATION

You will greet the candidate and record their candidate number and name and then hand over to the role player by saying:

> This is the trade union representative for a local construction team, who is also a construction worker. They will now start the station.

EXAMINER ANSWER GUIDANCE

The candidate should communicate clearly and accurately and provide reassurance that the risk posed by the human remains is extremely low and that the simple protective precautions recommended by the national health and safety regulator should provide perfectly adequate protection against the remote risk of exposure to potential infectious hazards. These measures should be taken in any case to protect against more likely environmental hazards such as lead dust, mould or parasite eggs on old coffin wood.

EXAMINER BRIEFING PACK

Marking guide for examiners

Specific marking guidance is carefully prepared to indicate to you when a candidate should fail (or excel) at a particular competency based on core material from the scenario. However, we recognise that we cannot anticipate all possible candidate responses. If a candidate says something that in your view merits a Grade E (or indicates excellence – Grade A) on that competency or station that we have not explicitly included in the marking guidance, it is important that you do then mark the candidate as a fail (or indicate excellence). In that situation, you need to operate outside the specific marking guidance, but please detail the issue in the examination feedback.

1. Has the candidate appropriately demonstrated *presenting skills* in a typical public health setting (presenting to a person or audience)?

Avoids jargon. Is clear. Appropriate language for the audience. Maintains eye contact. Appropriate manner for the situation. Shows empathy.

2. Has the candidate appropriately demonstrated *listening skills* in a typical public health setting (listening and responding appropriately)?

Ensures role player questions are answered appropriately. Answers totality of the question. Manner of response appropriate to role player scenario. Should not adopt an overly dismissive or patronising attitude toward the worker's concerns (marker of poor performance).

3. Has the candidate *demonstrated ascertainment of key public health facts from the material provided* and used it appropriately?

The candidate must present the following information, unprompted in a manner appropriate for the trade union official. Additional credit should be given to a clearly structured explanation.

GENERAL HAZARD

Infection hazards are very low from human cadavers that were buried many decades previously.

Cases of transmission of disease to those clearing burial grounds have not been documented even though many burial grounds have been cleared in recent years.

Old plague pits or charnel pits do not represent a significant hazard for infection with plague or other diseases.

Personal protection

Standard precautions should be taken against exposure to environmental biological hazards such as moulds and spores found in damp wood and earth, and lead-containing dust.

These measures should also provide adequate protection against the possible infection hazards of human cadavers that have been buried for a long period of time. These are the two key points for a good answer.

Specific hazards: microbiology

Only anthrax and smallpox represent a potential hazard, but the risk is very low in remains of this age (100–200 years) because:

Anthrax has been a relatively uncommon cause of death for the last 200 years, spore formation is only likely if there was significant blood contamination of the surrounding earth, and most healthy adults are moderately resistant to anthrax infection.

The evidence suggests that prolonged survival (more than 13 years) of infectious smallpox virus in non-living tissues does not occur.

Specific hazards: working environment

The risk of exposure to environmental biological hazards is likely to be greater for those working in enclosed spaces, such as crypts, than for those working in open burial grounds – excellent candidates might ask about the working conditions: Are they in enclosed spaces or out in the open?

The use of chloride of lime (quicklime) or other strong chemical disinfectants is not particularly effective and is likely to be hazardous to workers. Suggesting that chloride of lime or similar hazardous chemicals should be used to 'disinfect' the site is a marker of poor performance.

4. Has the candidate given a *balanced view* and/or *explained appropriately key public health concepts* in a public health setting?

An adequate answer requires the candidate to appreciate some of the wider aspects of construction work on a brownfield site. For example:

The candidate appreciates that there are lots of environmental hazards for construction workers and that adequate precautions are required against other biological and non-biological hazards; the cadavers are unlikely to be the greatest hazard.

Not mentioning the need for basic protective precautions against environmental hazards such as moulds, parasites and lead dust is a marker of poor performance.

The candidate appreciates that the union representative has another agenda (to increase the pay for his workers) but does not allow that to influence public health advice.

5. Has the candidate demonstrated sensitivity in handling *uncertainty, the unexpected, conflict* and/or *responding to challenging questions?*

The candidate explains clearly why the plague pit in one corner of the burial ground should not cause additional hazard.

The candidate appreciates the genuine concerns of the workforce, but is not persuaded by these concerns to provide overly cautious advice.

Agreeing that the work is too hazardous to be continued is a marker of poor performance.

Undermining the advice given by the national health and safety regulator is a fail criterion.

The candidate must maintain focus on the public health risks and on provision of evidence-based advice on appropriate precautions in the face of role players' attempts to use the situation to make the case for higher pay.

Role player briefing pack

STATION BACKGROUND

There is a major construction project to build a big shopping and entertainment complex in a run-down area of the large local town. The site for the new complex includes an old burial ground, which was in use throughout the nineteenth century and the early part of the twentieth century. The burial ground needs to be excavated and all the human remains removed, prior to putting in the foundations for the complex.

The senior trade union official for the construction workers at the site has asked for a meeting to discuss the possible hazards associated with clearing burial sites. He or she has already sought advice from the relevant national health and safety regulator. Neither he or she nor his members feel confident about the competence of the regulator to advise on a health issue such as this, and so now he or she wishes to get further assurance from the local public health (health protection) specialists.

BRIEFING ON BURIAL GROUND EXCAVATIONS AND INFECTION HAZARDS OF HUMAN REMAINS

Many old burial grounds are being cleared to allow foundations to be laid for new buildings. These excavations can involve removing coffins, some of which may be damaged or largely rotted away and some of which may be wholly intact. Some burial sites contain large pits where many bodies were buried together without coffins, often in successive layers, particularly at times of plague (which is a term used here for a particular type of infection called plague, rather than the more generic use of the term to describe any type of infection or infestation occurring in large numbers). Sometimes the whereabouts of plague pits were not recorded, and so they are found unexpectedly during the course of excavations.

Infectious diseases, such as tuberculosis, cholera, typhoid, plague, anthrax and smallpox, were much more common as causes of death in the nineteenth century than now (such diseases are now rare in this country), and therefore many people buried in graveyards dating from that period would have died of an infectious disease. Some of the organisms (bacteria and viruses) that cause these diseases can linger in and around the body of a dead person for a period of time after death, giving rise to concerns that dead bodies may be a source of infection for the living. For most organisms, however, this period of survival after a person's death is fairly short, and certainly there is no evidence of organisms surviving several years after burial.

The only infections for which there is some risk of survival for several years after death are smallpox (which causes a severe rash, high fever, and was often fatal) and anthrax (which is usually caught from working with infected animal hides and can cause either severe skin disease or a serious form of pneumonia that can be fatal).

MINIMISING THE RISKS OF INFECTION FROM HUMAN REMAINS THAT HAVE BEEN BURIED FOR A CENTURY OR MORE

For bodies that have been buried for several decades following death from anthrax or smallpox and certainly for those buried for 100 years or more, the risk that they may give rise to infection is very, very small. Even though these infections can be severe, the risk of catching infection from handling the bodies of those who died from either of these infections 100 years or more ago is considered to be negligible if simple precautions are taken when handling the remains, e.g. wearing face masks, gloves, overalls and protective glasses. This is largely because smallpox probably cannot survive more than a few years after death and because the conditions required for anthrax to survive for long periods are rarely found, and in any case most healthy people are moderately resistant to the infection.

There are other hazards associated with the work of clearing old burial sites that are likely to be a greater threat to the health of construction workers. These hazards include the mould found on old wooden coffins and in the surrounding earth, and lead dust from old lead coffins. Protective clothing, masks and glasses should be worn to protect against these hazards, and as noted above, this will also protect against any slight risk of exposure to infection from human remains. The risks associated with these other hazards, and the risk of exposure to any infectious material from human remains, are higher for people working in enclosed crypts than for those working on open burial grounds.

Quicklime, or chloride of lime, has been used in the past to disinfect mass burial sites, but there is no place for its use as a means of protecting against infection when excavating burial sites, not only because it is unlikely to be necessary or particularly effective, but more because it is a very hazardous substance in its own right that would pose a significant health risk to anyone working where it had been used.

The national health and safety regulator* is responsible for regulating safety on construction sites, and although they can provide health advice, unions are often keen to obtain independent local corroborating advice.

ROLE PLAYER BRIEF

You are a shop steward and senior area official for the major construction workers' trade union. You have a long history of working in the construction industry, having worked your way up from the bottom, and are proud of your achievements. You have a reputation for being a bit of a thorn in the side of the management.

You believe that the company that has been awarded the contract for the local construction work is not paying the construction staff enough for work that you feel is particularly hazardous.

You sought advice from the national health and safety regulator on the risks associated with graveyard clearances, but are sceptical about their expertise on health hazards and would like an independent opinion on their advice that basic standard precautions are all that is necessary.

What you know, but the candidate does not, is that the company has recently discovered old records indicating that there is a previously unknown plague pit at the site that is to be excavated, alongside the well-known burial ground. This information was given to the workforce yesterday, and this morning they have informed you that they are refusing to continue working on the site until they are provided with additional pay and protective clothing. They are expecting you to obtain support for this position from your discussions with the candidate.

Although you can be forthright and difficult with managers, you have some respect for health professionals and are likely to be moderately deferential to people such as the candidate. However, this respect and deferential attitude are likely to evaporate if you feel that you are being patronised or not being treated with due respect for your important position as an advocate for your members' interests. Become increasingly confident and pushy as the station progresses.

* The national health and safety regulator has the statutory duty to ensure companies abide by the relevant safety at work legislation. They have an enforcement and an advisory arm.

QUESTIONS

Your opening question should be:

> **Thanks for meeting me today. Is there much experience of this sort of thing? Wouldn't it be better to be safe than sorry?**
>
> [Candidate should give other environmental hazards as well as why infection is not a risk.]

Prompt by asking if there are risks other than infection if not mentioned, for example:

> **Are there other risks when we are digging up graves?**

If candidate doesn't say that there are no documented cases of transmission to workers in this situation, you may need prompt to ask:

> **Haven't other construction workers become ill after doing this sort of thing?**

Then introduce the new information about the plague pit:

Did you know there is an old plague pit where we are being asked to dig? They just showed me the records yesterday – surely this is a big risk to my workers?

[Expect explanation that the organism that causes plague is unlikely to survive long in a buried cadaver, even in mass burials such as plague pits, and these do not present a hazard.]

I know the national health and safety regulator said that we only need to wear masks, gloves and glasses with our overalls when we're digging up the graves, but that doesn't sound right to me, and it definitely can't be right if there's a plague pit there?

[Candidate should support national health and safety regulator advice, explaining that it deals with more likely environmental risks as well as remote risk of infection.]

I think we should be putting disinfectant or lime down, and fumigating the site – I read about them doing that when they had the big plague a few hundred years ago. You'd agree with that, wouldn't you?

[Candidate should explain why not to do this.]

This is dangerous work, we don't know what kind of things those people might have died of – my boys ought to be getting more pay for doing such a dangerous job, don't you agree? I mean, its not very comfortable wearing masks, and we only need to do it because of the risks we might get an infection from the dead bodies.

[Candidate should not get drawn into discussion of pay rates.]

ANY 'NO GO' AREAS

The candidate is not expected to cover issues relating to the legal framework for permissions, regulation or licensing of such excavations or to discuss the cultural or religious aspects.

LEVEL OF CONFLICT

The worker is in conflict with the employing construction company about rates of pay and is unhappy about the advice from the national health and safety regulator, and although he wants the candidate to give them some ammunition to take back to challenge both of these groups, he is not starting off with a sense of conflict with the candidate. However, he has a short fuse if he feels patronised or is not given due respect for his achievements and current position.

Blank Part B scenario feedback form

SCENARIO 1: INFECTION HAZARDS OF HUMAN CADAVERS

ACCESS AT http://goo.gl/IleQ7N

General performance

What was good?
What could be improved?

1. **Presenting communication** A B C D E

What was good?
What could be improved?

2. **Listening and comprehending** A B C D E

What was good?
What could be improved?

3. **Assimilating relevant information** A B C D E

What was good?
What could be improved?

4. **Reasoning, analytical and judgement** A B C D E

What was good?
What could be improved?

5. **Uncertainty and conflict** A B C D E

What was good?
What could be improved?

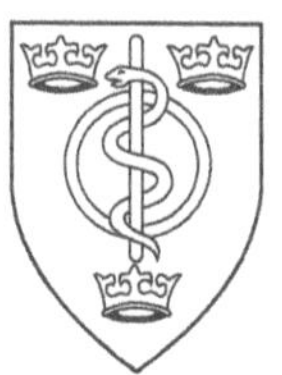

Faculty of Public Health

Of the Royal Colleges of Physicians of the United Kingdom

Working to improve the public's health

Scenario 2

Land contamination in a residential area

(original author Gerry Waldron, edited by Chris Packham and Jill Meara)

Candidate pack

CANDIDATE TASK

You are working in the public health department of your local health commissioning organisation.* You will meet with the chair of a local residents' group and brief him or her of your assessment of the risks to the health of the residents and what further actions (if any) are required to obtain further information.

You have 8 minutes to prepare for the station. You are not required to prepare any visual aids. You will then spend 8 minutes discussing the task with a role player. You may use paper notes to aid your verbal briefing.

OUTLINE OF SITUATION

A residential area within your locality was built in the late 1980s on a brownfield site† formerly occupied by a textile factory. Production ceased more than 25 years ago and the textile company is no longer in existence. Its assets are now owned by a large multinational corporation which, as a gesture of corporate responsibility, has informed the local council that it is concerned that the land might be heavily contaminated with high levels of carbon disulphide, which was extensively used in the manufacturing process. In 1985 the land was sold to a developer and subsequently to private homeowners, most of whom moved in from other districts and many of whom have lived in the area since. There are more than 200 dwellings in the development, none of which are built directly over the former factory area, which is located at the highest part of the site. A major investigation will be carried out over the next 3 months to determine the level of contamination in the land.

The residents have been informed of the situation. As a representative of the public health department the local council has asked for your help in determining the risks to the health of the residents in the area. The public health department has not been aware of any increased levels of ill health in the area, and the briefing pack contains some information from the census and the local cancer registry.

CANDIDATE GUIDANCE

You should begin by briefing the chair, focusing on the main risks, and then answer their questions, which will mainly centre on health risks to local residents and what should happen next.

AT THE STATION

You will be greeted by a marker examiner who will take your candidate number and name and then hand over to the role player by saying:

> This is the chair of the local residents' group. They will now start the station.

* A **primary care organisation** (PCO) is an NHS organisation that provides community and primary healthcare and commissions healthcare from community and hospital services. In England these are called primary care trusts (PCTs). A health board in Scotland performs some similar functions. PCTs and health boards generally cover designated areas and populations within those areas.

† A brownfield site is any land which has previously been used for any purpose and is no longer in use for that purpose. A site does not have to be contaminated, although contaminated land will automatically be brownfield.

CANDIDATE BRIEFING PACK

Item 1 From cancer registry to director of public health

Cancer registrations in the local housing development 1993–2003
16 persons diagnosed – 1 person had 2 tumours

3 non-melanoma skin cancers
3 breast
2 testis (a relatively rare tumour)
1 lung
1 oesophagus
1 prostate
1 kidney
1 ovary
1 leukaemia in a child
1 larynx
1 rectum

These are prevalence figures but work out at less than two new diagnoses per year (1993–2003).

We had done some calculations in the registry to estimate the number of cancers expected for different populations. If we have a population of 1000 people, we would expect 2 cancers per year, with the lower incidence of 1 per year and the upper of 10 per year without there being undue alarm. Lower and upper incidences for populations of 2000 had been calculated at 4 and 17 persons, respectively.

Item 2 From 2001 census – self-reported health status

Question	Area of the local development %	Locality %	District %	National %
Limiting long-term illness	13.8	23.3	22.8	25.6
General health				
Good health	78.4	70.4	70.9	70.0
Fairly good health	15.0	19.6	19.4	19.3
Not good health	6.6	10.1	9.7	10.7

Item 3 Briefing note on health effects of carbon disulphide

- **What are the contaminants?**
  The Department of the Environment has informed us that the possible contaminants on the site are carbon disulphide, sulphuric acid and various hydrocarbon compounds. Of these, the main chemical for possible concern is carbon disulphide.
- **What is carbon disulphide?**
  Carbon disulphide is a compound that is commonly used in the textile industry in the manufacture of rayon and other synthetic materials. In its physical state it is a colourless liquid with a characteristic odour.
- **What are the possible risks to health of carbon disulphide?**
  It should be emphasised that the most dangerous side effects of carbon

disulphide are seen when there is acute exposure to very large amounts such as chemical incidents/accidents, or with occupational exposure (effects on people who are directly handling and working with the chemicals for considerable periods of time). In these circumstances the effects of short-term exposure include irritation of the eyes, the skin and the respiratory tract. The substance may also affect the central nervous system.

In terms of long-term exposure in people working with the substance, there have been reports of skin conditions such as dermatitis, and effects on the cardiovascular and nervous system. Carbon disulphide is not believed to cause cancer in exposed individuals.

Examiner pack

EXAMINER SITUATION

You will greet the candidate and record their candidate number and name and then hand over to the role player by saying:

> This is the chair of the local residents' association. They will now start the station.

EXAMINER ANSWER GUIDANCE

The candidate is expected to be able to communicate approaches to describing the causation of disease, identify the characteristics of the local area, explain how prospective monitoring may be approached in this situation and describe the contribution health service public health teams can make in following up on residents' concerns. A detailed knowledge of the agencies and processes involved is not required.

EXAMINER BRIEFING PACK

Marking guide for examiners

1. Has the candidate appropriately demonstrated *presenting skills* in a typical public health setting (presenting to a person or audience)?

   > Avoids jargon. Is clear. Appropriate language for the audience. Maintains eye contact. Appropriate manner for the situation. Shows empathy.

2. Has the candidate appropriately demonstrated *listening skills* in a typical public health setting (listening and responding appropriately)?

   > Ensures role player questions are answered appropriately. Answers totality of the question. Manner of response appropriate to role player scenario.

3. Has the candidate *demonstrated ascertainment of key public health facts from the material provided* and used it appropriately?

   > Risks inherent in geographical location of site, downhill and possibly downstream from old factory site.
   >
   > Facts on carbon disulphide – occupational versus environmental exposure risks – not always possible to extrapolate from one to the other.
   >
   > Health of local population compared with local/national picture – lower levels of ill health than surrounding population, lower cancer incidence, higher socio-economic profile.
   >
   > Lack of evidence of increased ill health not necessarily proof that risk is absent.

4. Has the candidate given a *balanced view* and/or *explained appropriately key public health concepts* in a public health setting?

   > Puts information in context of limited knowledge of environmental risk.
   >
   > Points out long history of habitation on site without apparent ill effects.
   >
   > Discusses multi-factorial causation of conditions such as cancer, heart disease, etc.
   >
   > Recognises that mental distress over the situation may in itself be a direct or indirect contributory factor in future ill health.

5. Has the candidate demonstrated sensitivity in handling *uncertainty, the unexpected, conflict* and/or *responding to challenging questions?*

Sensitive and empathic to real concerns of residents and the uncertain situation in which they find themselves.

Mentions uncertainty in relation to environmental effects, level of contaminant (if any) present on site.

Keeps to health remit, recognising that property values and possible litigation issues are best dealt with by other agencies.

Outlines role of public health department in following up on information from investigation and taking necessary action, working with local and national partners, e.g. council, Health Protection Agency (HPA)* (Chemical Hazards and Poisons Division). Specifically outlines what happens next and a commitment to keep the residents informed and offer contact details and a timetable of next steps.

* A **HPA** is a national body of experts who advise healthcare organisations and others on public heath protection issues around infectious and environmental hazards.

Role player briefing pack

STATION BACKGROUND

As candidate briefing.

ROLE PLAYER BRIEF

You are the chair of the local residents' association and have lived in the area for 15 years. You are concerned about the effect on the value of your house, but more importantly about possible adverse health effects. You are aware of two local people who have died of cancer in the past 5 years – one had a brain tumour and another lung cancer. Your son looked up carbon disulphide on the Internet and told you that it causes 'nerve and heart damage'.

Start the meeting by introducing yourself and prompting the candidate to begin:

> **Thanks very much for agreeing to meet with me. We are all very worried about this situation. How big a risk is there to our health?**

Depending on the initial summary ask:

> **Well what do the local statistics tell us?**

At the earliest opportunity raise the issue of your two neighbours with cancer. Ask:

> **Is there a connection between the two cases of cancer in my neighbours?**
>
> **What are you going to do to monitor the situation?**
>
> **They must have known about this for years – why weren't we told anything?**

Before the end of the station ask:

> **What about property values – who is responsible for compensating the residents for physical and mental distress?**

ANY 'NO GO' AREAS

Do not discuss complex toxicological or clinical issues. If candidate raises these say, 'I'm just an ordinary person. What's the bottom line here?'

LEVEL OF CONFLICT

High at first, in keeping with level of anxiety about situation. If candidate addresses concerns appropriately, conflict level lowered to reflect this. Maintain high level of suspicion about government and multinationals.

Blank Part B scenario feedback form

SCENARIO 2: LAND CONTAMINATION IN A RESIDENTIAL AREA

ACCESS AT http://goo.gl/ubPL7y

General performance

What was good?
What could be improved?

1. **Presenting communication** A B C D E

What was good?
What could be improved?

2. **Listening and comprehending** A B C D E

What was good?
What could be improved?

3. **Assimilating relevant information** A B C D E

What was good?
What could be improved?

4. **Reasoning, analytical and judgement** A B C D E

What was good?
What could be improved?

5. **Uncertainty and conflict** A B C D E

What was good?
What could be improved?

Faculty of Public Health

Of the Royal Colleges of Physicians of the United Kingdom

Working to improve the public's health

Scenario 3

Human papilloma virus (HPV) vaccine to prevent cervical cancer

(original author Linda Garvican, edited by Chris Packham and Jill Meara)

Candidate pack

CANDIDATE TASK

You are a member of the public health team in a primary care organisation* serving a population of 500,000 people which is in financial deficit. You have been asked to provide a verbal briefing to the chair of the local clinical advisory committee,† who is also a general practitioner (GP), to assist the chair in some early informal discussions with their colleague general practitioners (later today) to help decide how the PCO will handle provision of this vaccine.

You have 8 minutes to prepare for the station. You are not required to prepare any visual aids. You will then spend 2–3 minutes summarising the situation and the remainder of the time discussing the task with a role player. You may use paper notes to aid your verbal briefing.

OUTLINE OF SITUATION

Cervical cancer is strongly associated with persistent infection with human papilloma virus (HPV). Two vaccines against HPV are licensed. The Joint Committee on Vaccinations and Immunisations‡ (JCVI) is recommending that vaccination is given to girls aged 12–13 and the Department of Health has agreed to support the programme 'in principle'.

However, there is to be a review of cost-effectiveness, and the programme is expected to start in September 2008. Public interest has been re-awakened by the media, and some GPs have been receiving requests from parents. Some want to be able to prescribe it for young women and girls in their practices now, but you have also heard about some opposition from faith groups.

There are less than 40 cases of cervical cancer each year in your PCO area – audit data suggests that the majority of cases are in women who have either never been screened or have not taken up screening for at least 5 years. Coverage of cervical screening in the area is 85%. There are around 2500 girls in each school year group within your PCO population. Your department has prepared some briefing notes (candidate pack) which the chair has also received.

CANDIDATE GUIDANCE

- Brief the chair on the factual information about the vaccine and the proposed immunisation programme.
- Discuss the implications for the local screening programme.

* A **primary care organisation** (PCO) is an NHS organisation that provides community and primary healthcare and commissions healthcare from community and hospital services. In England these are called primary care trusts (PCTs). A health board in Scotland performs some similar functions. PCTs and health boards generally cover designated areas and populations within those areas.

† A committee which provides professional clinical advice on behalf of primary care within the primary care organisation.

‡ Vaccination policy in the UK is determined by the Joint Committee on Vaccinations and Immunisations (JCVI) of the Department of Health.

AT THE STATION

You will be greeted by a marker examiner who will take your candidate number and name and then hand over to the role player by saying:

> This is the chair of our committee. They will now start the station.

CANDIDATE BRIEFING PACK

Edited extracts:

1. **Cervical Screening Programme Regional Quality Assurance Reference Centre position statement on vaccination to prevent cervical cancer: March 2007**

   1.1. **Cervical Cancer in this area**

   Ninety-nine percent of specimens of cervical carcinoma contain human papilloma virus (HPV). Two of these, HPV types 16 and 18, are believed to cause about 70% of cervical cancer. Precancerous cellular changes or lesions preceding cervical cancer can be diagnosed by histology. They are known as cervical intraepithelial neoplasia (CIN). CIN is graded 1, 2 or 3, with the higher numbers representing higher-grade lesions.

   1.2. **Prevention of cervical cancer**

   Screening The UK national cervical cytology screening programme prevents 80% of cases of cervical cancer.

   Vaccine A vaccine to prevent cervical cancer has recently been licensed. This protects against HPV strains 16 and 18 and also two other strains, 6 and 11, which are known to cause genital warts. The vaccine is administered in three doses over a period of 3 months and the course costs about £240 per patient. Studies on one vaccine were carried out in young women aged 16–26 with a maximum follow-up of 5 years. Three doses were shown to be effective in preventing CIN development in those who had not been exposed to HPV and the vaccine was well tolerated. There is as yet no evidence that the vaccine provides lifelong immunity.

   There is a possibility that other strains of HPV will become dominant in vaccinated populations, and there will be many women at risk of cervical cancer for many years to come, so that cervical screening is still required for the foreseeable future.

   1.3. **National policy**

   The JCVI has supported the use of the vaccine in girls as outlined below. The government will fund the supply of vaccine though not administration costs. The American equivalent of the JCVI has already recommended that young girls should indeed be vaccinated but has not provided the funding. Several other countries are also recommending its use. The cost-benefit analysis carried out was favourable but very sensitive to changes in cost assumptions.

   1.4. **Present situation**

   Current advice is to await national guidance. The licensed vaccines may be legally prescribed. PCOs need to discourage individual GPs prescribing it on the National Health Service (NHS) in an ad hoc and uncoordinated manner. A JCVI meeting in June 2007 concluded:

   - HPV vaccines should be introduced routinely for girls aged around 12–13 years, subject to independent peer review of the cost-benefit analysis.
   - An additional cost-effectiveness analysis to determine the benefits of a catch-up for older girls was required before a recommendation could be made by the main committee.
   - Any new data on HPV vaccines would be kept under review by JCVI.

2. **Summary of evidence of effectiveness of one of the vaccines**

   The FUTURE II Study Group, Quadrivalent vaccine against human papillomavirus to prevent high-grade cervical lesions, *New England Journal of Medicine* 356, 1915–1927, 2007.

Randomised, double-blind trial, 12,167 women aged 15–26 years, randomised to receive three doses of either HPV vaccine or placebo, administered at day 1, month 2 and month 6.

The primary composite end point was the development of cervical intraepithelial neoplasia (CIN) grade 2 or 3, or adenocarcinoma *in situ*, or cervical cancer related to HPV-16 or HPV-18.

Subjects were followed for an average of 3 years after receiving the first dose. There were no cases of cervical cancer in either group during follow-up, and numbers of adenocarcinoma *in situ* were too small to show statistically significant differences. However, there were substantial numbers of new cases of CIN as the main component of the primary composite end point.

In the vaccine group ($n = 6087$), there was 1 possible HPV-16/18-associated CIN, while in the placebo group ($n = 6080$) there were 42 such lesions detected.

Vaccine efficacies for the prevention of the primary composite end point were

- 98% (95% confidence interval [CI], 86–100) in the susceptible population with no evidence of infection with HPV-16 or HPV-18 until after completion of the three-dose immunisation
- 44% (95% CI, 26–58) in an intention-to-treat population of all randomised women (those with or without previous infection)

The authors concluded that in young women who had not been previously infected with HPV-16 or HPV-18, those in the vaccine group had a significantly lower occurrence of high-grade CIN related to HPV-16 or HPV-18 than did those in the placebo group.

Examiner pack

EXAMINER SITUATION

You will greet the candidate and record their candidate number and name and then hand over to the role player by saying:

> This is the chair of the committee. They will now start the station.

EXAMINER ANSWER GUIDANCE

This question is a mixture of appraisal of summary evidence and assessment of a practical situation, where public health advice is needed to ensure that health funds and professional efforts are not spent in an ineffective or uncoordinated manner, despite the appearance that this intervention is a good thing. Some issues such as quality control of advice given as part of the vaccination process and cost-effectiveness are not presented in briefing material as they remain to be finalised and are areas of uncertainty candidates should recognise. The candidate will be expected to demonstrate good listening skills to the GP's questions.

EXAMINER BRIEFING PACK

Marking guide for examiners

1. Has the candidate appropriately demonstrated *presenting skills* in a typical public health setting (presenting to a person or audience)?

Avoids jargon. Is clear. Appropriate language for the audience. Maintains eye contact. Appropriate manner for the situation. Shows empathy.

2. Has the candidate appropriately demonstrated *listening skills* in a typical public health setting (listening and responding appropriately)?

Ensures role player questions are answered appropriately. Answers totality of the question. Manner of response appropriate to role player scenario – recognises pressure on GPs from parents and teenage girls.

3. Has the candidate *demonstrated ascertainment of key public health facts from the material provided* and used it appropriately?

> Understood and presented back summary of case accurately, interpreted facts and data from the research study accurately, and explained the evidence from the study, identifying that the findings are unlikely to be due to chance. Key issues appropriately stressed:
>
> - Effectiveness best pre-exposure
> - Need for cervical screening will remain (long period of already exposed and at-risk women)
> - Potential for shift in HPV types implicated in cervical cancer aetiology
> - As yet unclear as to potential effects, if any, on risk-taking behaviour around sexually transmitted infections and messages taken by teenagers
>
> Recognised this is fairly rare cancer. Explained epidemiological terms simply to chair.

4. Has the candidate given a *balanced view* and/or *explained appropriately key public health concepts* in a public health setting?

> Understood and explained public health concepts accurately and in an appropriate manner for the chair including issues around ensuring potential equity of access and uptake challenges. Good candidates should be able to explain the concept of opportunity costs, and there are other options to spend this money.
>
> Good candidates will also mention training implications, advice for parents and girls, use of school nursing resources, media handling issues, especially around ethical concerns, and potential use of media to dispel potential myths (e.g. vaccine against STIs).

5. Has the candidate demonstrated sensitivity in handling *uncertainty, the unexpected, conflict* and/or *responding to challenging questions?*

Non-confrontational, ensures balanced view, acknowledges uncertainty. Candidate should be able to handle the uncertainty and sympathise with the GPs but be clear that the decision should be made on the evidence of effectiveness. Good candidates will identify ongoing uncertainties such as potential effects on risk-taking behaviour and longer-term effectiveness issues.

Role player briefing pack

STATION BACKGROUND

As candidate briefing.

ROLE PLAYER BRIEF

You are the chair of your clinical advisory committee, in a PCO which is in financial deficit, and your committee is due to meet later today to discuss the possible provision of a vaccine to prevent cervical cancer. You have asked for a briefing with the representative of the public health department before the meeting to summarise and clarify the position and to help develop a clear message for local GPs. The public health representative will give a 2- to 3-minute verbal briefing followed by discussion and questions from you.

The committee has to discuss this issue and make recommendations to the PCO on how to handle the provision of this vaccine. Many of your fellow GPs have had several requests from concerned affluent parents who want this vaccine to be provided now for their teenage daughters.

ROLE PLAYER SCRIPT

Thank you for coming to see me. I've only read this briefly, so can you please summarise what is being recommended. I'm meeting my GP colleagues later today.

If the candidate does not explain what the data means:

So what is the evidence showing and what does 'vaccine efficacy' actually mean?

Why can't we implement this now?

How much will the vaccination programme reduce cervical cancer?

Ask:

Can you be sure? By when?

If the candidate seems unsure or does not give a clear explanation:

How are we going to make sure everyone who needs this gets it – especially in the more deprived areas?

[Press the candidates if they do not offer any potential methods of implementing the programme and trying to ensure equity of access, e.g. via GPs, via school nurses etc.]

Unless covered:

So will we be stopping cervical screening soon?

To sum up:

So what would you recommend we do at this point?

ANY 'NO GO' AREAS

Details of evaluation of the vaccine efficacy beyond that in the evidence presented.

LEVEL OF CONFLICT

Medium.

Blank Part B scenario feedback form

SCENARIO 3: HPV VACCINE TO PREVENT CERVICAL CANCER

ACCESS AT http://goo.gl/omN5tF

General performance

What was good?
What could be improved?

1. **Presenting communication** A B C D E

What was good?
What could be improved?

2. **Listening and comprehending** A B C D E

What was good?
What could be improved?

3. **Assimilating relevant information** A B C D E

What was good?
What could be improved?

4. **Reasoning, analytical and judgement** A B C D E

What was good?
What could be improved?

5. **Uncertainty and conflict** A B C D E

What was good?
What could be improved?

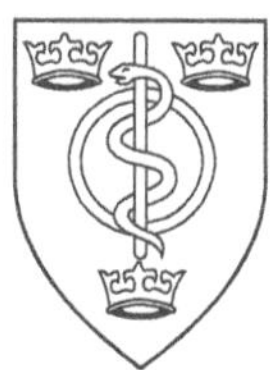

Faculty of Public Health

Of the Royal Colleges of Physicians of the United Kingdom

Working to improve the public's health

Scenario 4

Interview on speed cameras

(original author Christine Hine, edited by Chris Packham and Jill Meara)

Candidate pack

CANDIDATE TASK

You are a member of a public health department in a local health organisation. A journalist from your local newspaper wants to interview you. The interview will be on local use of speed cameras.* They want to speak to you on the telephone.

You have 8 minutes to prepare for the station. You are not required to prepare any visual aids. You will then spend 8 minutes being interviewed by a role player. You may use paper notes during the interview.

OUTLINE OF SITUATION

The journalist wants to speak to you on the telephone as they are doing an article for the local newspaper on speed cameras and need to have the article ready in the next few hours. You know that speed cameras have been in the news again since their use was supported as part of the local road safety strategy. You have been briefed by a colleague who had worked on the road safety strategy partnership, but they are not available. The key elements of the local strategy were

- Improving safety for children – especially as pedestrians and cyclists
- Promoting safe use of vulnerable transport modes – walking, cycling, motorcycling and horse riding
- Reducing excessive and inappropriate speed of motor vehicles (including promoting the use of speed cameras)
- Targeting other poor driving practices – use of mobile phones, drink driving, drug driving and driving while tired

The communications department in your organisation has set up the interview in response to a request from the journalist. They are under the impression that the journalist dislikes speed cameras.

CANDIDATE GUIDANCE

You do not know what the journalist is going to ask you. Prepare possible responses so that you can present a balanced view of the advantages and disadvantages of speed cameras in the local context, using evidence you have available at the time (briefing pack).

AT THE STATION

You will be greeted by a marker examiner who will take your candidate number and name, and then you will be asked to start the telephone conversation with:

> Please sit down and wait for the telephone call from the journalist [which will be carried out by a role player]. This will start the station.

* A **speed camera** is a roadside camera which is triggered by cars that exceed the speed limit, enabling the police to use the photographs as evidence if they choose to prosecute.

CANDIDATE BRIEFING PACK

Evidence and arguments for use of speed cameras

1. **Information from Parliamentary Advisory Council for Transport Safety (PACTS) and the Slower Speeds Initiative (SSI), Speed cameras: Criticisms and why they are flawed, research briefing, December 2003**

   Crash investigations show excessive or inappropriate speed is a major contributory factor in at least one-third of all road crashes the single most important contributory factor to road casualties. Even slight decreases in speed are beneficial. When the U.S. national speed limit was lowered to 55 mph, fatality rates dropped by 50% on the interstate highways and by 70% on other four-lane rural highways.

   A 'poll of polls' by Transport 2000 (a pressure group) – based on six different surveys – shows that support for the use of speed cameras averages 74%.

   Government criteria must be satisfied before a new camera can be installed. There must have been at least four deaths or serious injuries on a given 1.5 km stretch of road within the past 3 years. At least 20% of drivers must be exceeding the speed limit, 'and there are no other obvious, practical measures to improve road safety along this stretch of road'.

   The study indicated that the drivers most likely to be caught on camera (company car drivers and drivers with high mileage) were more likely to have a speeding conviction and more likely to be involved in crashes than other drivers. Company car drivers and high-mileage drivers who drive for work are 50% more likely to be involved in injury accidents than other drivers, even after differences in exposure due to miles driven have been taken into account.

   There is no logical reason or evidence to suggest speed cameras are responsible for a decline in the rate of reduction of road casualties. Great reductions were seen in the 1980s at the time when compulsory use of front seat belts was introduced, car design improved and drink driving fatalities reduced. More recently, however, traffic has increased, drink driving fatalities have levelled off, seat belt wearing has declined and use of mobile phones while driving has increased.

   In a 2-year pilot study of cameras in six counties, 280 fewer people were killed or seriously injured at camera sites than expected. The total cost saving of casualties at camera sites over 2 years was around £58 million, several times higher than both the amount spent on camera enforcement (£21 million) and the amount raised in fixed penalty income (£27 million). Taking account of reduction in casualties, the total estimated benefit to society over 2 years was approximately £112 million. A previous cost-benefit analysis of speed cameras found that cameras generate a return of five times the investment after 1 year and 25 times the amount after 5 years. Neither the police nor local authorities retain income from speed cameras.

   PACTS and SSI believe that identifying road traffic enforcement and casualty reduction as a key policing priority would have a major effect in reversing the decline of traffic policing.

   There is no evidence of speed cameras causing a reduction in the number of serious offences detected. Dangerous driving offences recorded between 1998–1999 and 2002–2003 showed an increase.

2. **Findings of Pilkington P and Kinra S, Effectiveness of speed cameras in preventing road traffic collisions and related casualties: Systematic review, *BMJ*, 330, 331–334, 2005**

   The main outcome measures considered were road traffic collisions, injuries and deaths. Controlled trials and observational studies assessing the impact of fixed or mobile speed cameras on any of the selected outcomes were included. Fourteen observational studies met the inclusion criteria; no randomised controlled trials were found. Most studies were before-after studies without controls ($n = 8$). All but one of the studies showed effectiveness of cameras up to 3 years or less after their introduction; one study showed sustained longer-term effects (4.6 years after introduction).

Reductions in outcomes across studies ranged from 5% to 69% for collisions, 12% to 65% for injuries, and 17% to 71% for deaths in the immediate vicinity of camera sites. **The authors concluded that existing research consistently shows speed cameras are an effective intervention in reducing road traffic collisions and related casualties.** The level of evidence is relatively poor, however, as most studies did not have satisfactory comparison groups or adequate control for potential confounders. Controlled introduction of speed cameras with careful data collection may offer improved evidence of their effectiveness in the future.

3. **Local profile of the area**

   You work in an area of average deprivation and morbidity for the country but with a very high rate of road traffic accidents in children and in older people (79 killed or seriously injured per 100,000 compared with a regional average of 59 for the most recent year available). These accidents also were much more common in more deprived communities within your area. There has been pressure to act on this for some time, mainly focused on improving road links and the construction of a new bypass around one urban area. However, these changes are some years away and action is needed now to reduce deaths.

Examiner pack

EXAMINER SITUATION

You will greet the candidate and record their candidate number and name and then hand over to the role player by saying

> Please sit down and wait for the telephone call from the journalist [which will be carried out by a role player]. This will start the station.

EXAMINER ANSWER GUIDANCE

Criticism and dislike of speed cameras is commonly expressed in the media and on websites. The briefing pack sets out arguments in their favour and findings from one systematic review (which provoked a large and mixed set of rapid responses when published in the *BMJ*).

In providing a balanced public health view, the candidate should:

- Acknowledge the body of evidence supporting use of speed cameras to enforce speed control, and provide examples
- Demonstrate awareness of the limitations of the evidence, and the problem of limited acceptability to the public
- Be clear that speed control is a necessary part of road safety strategy

On the basis of the information in the briefing pack, it would not be acceptable for a candidate to support the view that evidence and arguments are so weak as to seriously question the use of speed cameras.

If the candidate acknowledges supporting evidence but goes on to cite further evidence against speed cameras, the examiner should make a judgement of the credibility and appropriateness of the overall view given and mark accordingly.

Candidates putting forward a negative view must still cover the brief given in this scenario, i.e. competently present evidence **for** speed cameras, whatever else they may want to add.

EXAMINER BRIEFING PACK

Marking guide for examiners

1. Has the candidate appropriately demonstrated *presenting skills* in a typical public health setting (presenting to a person or audience)?

> Avoids jargon. Is clear. Appropriate language for the audience. Maintains eye contact. Appropriate manner for the situation. Shows empathy.

2. Has the candidate appropriately demonstrated *listening skills* in a typical public health setting (listening and responding appropriately)?

> Ensures role player questions are answered appropriately. Answers totality of the question. Manner of response appropriate to role player scenario.

3. Has the candidate demonstrated ascertainment of key public health facts from the material provided and used it appropriately?

> Identifies that use of cameras is only one part of road safety strategy, noting examples of other strategic aims listed in the 'outline of situation'.
>
> Uses examples from the briefing pack to convey that there is good supporting evidence for speed cameras, while acknowledging limitations. (Examples of limitations could include methodological weaknesses of before and after studies, and difficulties of attributing favourable trends in road safety statistics to single interventions. There are many suitable examples of supporting evidence provided in the briefing pack.)

4. Has the candidate given a *balanced view* and/or *explained appropriately key public health concepts* in a public health setting?

A balanced view would feature the following elements:

- The body of evidence supporting use of speed cameras to enforce speed control is substantial, albeit that there are limitations. Further research may help.
- Limited acceptability to the public is an issue, but there is evidence from polls of public support.
- An unequivocal view that speed control is a necessary part of road safety strategy.

An acceptable performance must include and promote in the time available other key issues, such as:

- Targeting poor driving practices (use of mobile phones, drink/drug driving, and driving while tired)
- Improving safety for children (role of structural alterations including cycle routes and speed)
- Restriction methods, etc.
- Promoting safe use of vulnerable transport modes – walking, cycling

5. Has the candidate demonstrated sensitivity in handling *uncertainty, the unexpected, conflict* and/or *responding to challenging questions?*

Candidate responds calmly to the journalist's attempts to undermine local road safety strategy. Candidate is not deflected from the task of conveying key public health points. Candidate ensures that all aspects of the question guidance are covered in the time available. Poor candidates will fail to do this.

Role player briefing pack

STATION BACKGROUND

You are a journalist working for a local newspaper. Since a speed camera was installed on one of the roads leading to your office, you and several colleagues have been fined for breaking the 30 mph speed limit. The general opinion at your workplace is that the road was safe and the only reason for installing a camera was to make money from fining motorists who were not doing any harm. The editor has given you the opportunity to work up a feature for the paper on what really lies behind local use of speed cameras.

The local authority road safety strategy was produced by a partnership 2 years ago, which included a member from the local department of public health who advised on evidence of health benefits related to road safety measures. You try to contact this person, but they have moved to a new post. Instead you are offered a telephone interview to discuss speed cameras with a public health department team member who was not involved in developing the strategy.

ROLE PLAYER BRIEF

Start the interview by introducing yourself and explaining what you are doing:

> **Thanks for talking to me. I'm putting together a feature on speed cameras for the paper. I understand you can tell me a bit about why we should have to put up with having speed cameras all over the place.**

This should prompt the candidate to start by explaining that speed cameras can help in enforcing speed control, an important element of road safety strategy. They should also note the other elements of the strategy (listed in their pack). If not, prompt them by asking:

> **Surely there is more to road safety than just putting speed cameras up?**

Depending on what the candidate has covered already, continue to focus on the camera issue in the interview. A good candidate will want to start discussing the other measures in the strategy. You might continue to try and cover the following but should pick up on the other issues if they are mentioned (driver skill, alternative transport, etc.).

> **Cameras could be causing more accidents, because they make people suddenly brake hard. How can you be sure that they are not doing more harm than good?**
>
> [Prompt the candidate to go into some detail on the evidence: 'Just how good is this evidence?' 'How do you know that any changes in numbers of accidents are due to cameras rather than other things that influence the ways people drive?']
>
> **Some of us think that cameras are actually catching safe drivers barely exceeding the speed limit rather than much younger men who are most likely to cause major accidents. How do you know they are catching the right people?**
>
> **It looks like cameras are set up in places that will make the most money rather than in the most dangerous places. What do you think?**
>
> **One thing that really annoys people is that the limits are set too low. It would not be so bad having speed cameras if they were set at say 40 mph rather than 30 mph in residential areas. Why can't the local authority be more receptive to what the public wants – faster roads and fewer cameras?**

No later than the '1 minute to go' bell, ask the candidate the following question:

> **So please summarise what you feel are the most important issues in helping to reduce road deaths?**
>
> **Will we be scrapping speed cameras?**

ANY 'NO GO' AREAS

The candidate is not expected to have any knowledge of debates that might have gone on at the time the local authority strategy was agreed.

LEVEL OF CONFLICT

You are still annoyed at having been fined for speeding and can see no benefits in having speed cameras on roads like the one you were caught on. You expect that the feature you are preparing for the paper will not be supportive of speed cameras. You will be calm but focused in trying to undermine any good news on the value of speed cameras.

Blank Part B scenario feedback form

SCENARIO 4: INTERVIEW ON SPEED CAMERAS

ACCESS AT Access at http://goo.gl/83R0Hb

General performance

What was good?
What could be improved?

1. **Presenting communication** A B C D E

What was good?
What could be improved?

2. **Listening and comprehending** A B C D E

What was good?
What could be improved?

3. **Assimilating relevant information** A B C D E

What was good?
What could be improved?

4. **Reasoning, analytical and judgement** A B C D E

What was good?
What could be improved?

5. **Uncertainty and conflict** A B C D E

What was good?
What could be improved?

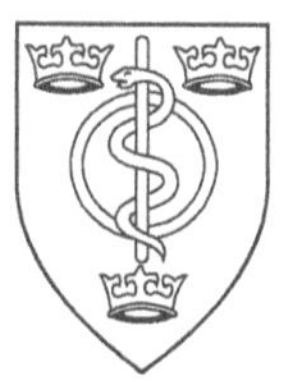

Faculty of Public Health

Of the Royal Colleges of Physicians of the United Kingdom

Working to improve the public's health

Scenario 5

Exceptional funding request

(original author Adrian Mairs, edited by Chris Packham and Jill Meara)

Candidate pack

CANDIDATE TASK

The director of public health (DPH) has just phoned and asked you to come to see him or her about a request for funding for an anti-cancer drug called erlotinib for a patient – Mrs Smith.

You have 8 minutes to prepare for the station. You are not required to prepare any visual aids. You will then spend 2–3 minutes giving a verbal presentation, and there will then be discussion with the role player for the remainder of the 8-minute scenario. You may use paper notes to aid your verbal briefing.

OUTLINE OF SITUATION

You are a public health trainee. In your organisation there is a 'specialist medicines group' which is multidisciplinary and considers requests for funding for individuals for high-cost drugs not normally available in the healthcare system. It meets monthly. The DPH is not a member of the group. Your consultant trainer is a member but is on leave. They have left you a briefing (enclosed items 1 and 2) about a recent decision on a patient that might require further work while they are away.

Erlotinib is licensed for the treatment of patients with locally advanced, or metastatic, non-small-cell lung cancer (NSCLC), in whom at least one prior chemotherapy regimen has failed. National Institute* guidance on the use of erlotinib within the health service is attached (**Item 1**). In addition, there is some evidence that erlotinib is more effective in females, in non-smokers and in a type of NSCLC called bronchioloalveolar carcinoma (BAC). This type of lung cancer is relatively rare (5% of all lung cancers) and tends to occur in younger, non-smoking females.

Mrs Smith has BAC and is a non-smoker. She is 58 and has had four cycles of chemotherapy with gemcitabine and carboplatin (both alternative chemotherapeutic agents). This was followed with docetaxel due to disease progression. Further disease progression resulted in her being treated with erlotinib, which she is funding herself. She has been taking erlotinib for more than a year now and her disease has remained stable.

At a recent meeting the group considered a request for funding for erlotinib for Mrs Smith. The request described the type of patients that might benefit from erlotinib and pointed out that Mrs Smith matched this profile. However, it did

* A **national institute** is a national body of clinical experts responsible for assessing the effectiveness of medical technologies. In England it is referred to as the National Institute for Health and Clinical Excellence (NICE). In other European countries it may be called a national advisory body. The guidance issued by this body is used to plan and fund largely new and expensive technologies within the healthcare system.

not mention any other 'exceptional' factors* and the funding request was rejected (letter attached: **Item 2**). Your healthcare organisation is under considerable financial pressure at the moment and the number of requests for high-cost drugs is rising.

CANDIDATE GUIDANCE

There has been a lot of recent media coverage about patients who have been denied anti-cancer medicines, including a recent television programme which showed that some healthcare organisations approved most requests on the basis of exceptionality, whereas others approved very few. You suspect that this is why the DPH wants to speak to you.

You should be prepared to brief the DPH as far as possible from the briefing material and your knowledge of prioritisation issues in the healthcare system. The DPH has the briefing material.

AT THE STATION

You will be greeted by a marker examiner who will take your candidate number and name and then hand over to the role player by saying:

> This is the Director of Public Health. They will now start the station.

Candidate briefing pack: Item 1

National institute for health and clinical excellence

FINAL APPRAISAL DETERMINATION

Erlotinib for the treatment of non-small-cell lung cancer

1. Guidance
   1.1. Erlotinib is recommended, within its licensed indication, as an alternative to docetaxel as a second-line treatment option for patients with non-small-cell lung cancer (NSCLC) only on the basis that it is provided by the manufacturer at an overall treatment cost equal to that of docetaxel.
   1.2. Erlotinib is not recommended for the second-line treatment of locally advanced or metastatic NSCLC in patients for whom docetaxel is unsuitable (i.e. where there is intolerance of or contraindications to docetaxel) or for third-line treatment after docetaxel therapy.
   1.3. People currently receiving treatment with erlotinib, but for whom treatment would not be recommended according to Section 1.2, should have the option to continue treatment until they and their clinicians consider it appropriate to stop.

Issue date: September 2008

* Exceptional factors were required to justify a funding request in this scenario. These relate to a patient's ability to benefit more than average clinically due to individual physical factors that predicted (using evidence) a particularly favourable response.

Candidate briefing pack: Item 2

LETTER FROM THE SPECIALIST MEDICINES GROUP TO THE CLINICIAN REQUESTING FUNDING FOR ERLOTINIB

Thank you for your letter. You are seeking funding to treat this patient with erlotinib, as a third-line treatment for bronchioloalveolar carcinoma (BAC) on the basis that she is an exceptional case.

For a patient to be considered exceptional he or she should be:

- Different from the general population of patients with the condition in question
- Likely to gain significantly more benefit from the intervention than might be expected from the average patient with the condition

The fact that a patient's clinical condition matches the accepted indications for a treatment that is not routinely funded is not in itself sufficient for that case to be considered exceptional. Social value judgements are rarely relevant to the consideration of exceptional status.

From the information available, it appears that this woman is part of a subgroup of patients with non-small-cell lung cancer that may achieve a survival advantage from third-line treatment with erlotinib. The implication is that you would put forward all such patients to be considered for this treatment. If that is the case, then it follows that they are not being put forward as individual exceptions, but as members of a subgroup who may benefit from a particular treatment.

This therefore appears to be a service development issue, applicable to several patients meeting the same clinical criteria and as such it is not appropriate for consideration through the exceptional case process. I regret therefore that we are not in a position to fund this treatment.

Yours sincerely,
Chair of the Specialist Medicines Group

Examiner pack

EXAMINER SITUATION

You will greet the candidate and record their candidate number and name and then hand over to the role player by saying:

> This is the Director of Public Health. They will now start the station.

EXAMINER ANSWER GUIDANCE

This is a common situation for some service public health specialists in the NHS. Candidates may not be familiar with all the details contained in the scenario, but should be aware of the main issues around prioritisation and be able to sensibly respond to the questions posed. Good candidates will be more aware of some of the subtleties contained in the question, e.g. the issue of individual exceptional (appropriate for such a funding group) versus a subset that indicate a significant population need, requiring a service development for all patients with similar demographic and pathological indicators of prognosis. All candidates should be able to identify the basic facts around prognosis and link this to the subject of the scenario to pass. A balanced and objective approach is also required to pass.

EXAMINER BRIEFING PACK

Marking guide for examiners

1. Has the candidate appropriately demonstrated *presenting skills* in a typical public health setting (presenting to a person or audience)?

> Avoids jargon. Is clear. Appropriate language for the audience. Maintains eye contact. Appropriate manner for the situation. Shows empathy.

2. Has the candidate appropriately demonstrated *listening skills* in a typical public health setting (listening and responding appropriately)?

> Ensures role player questions are answered appropriately. Answers totality of the question. Manner of response appropriate to role player scenario.

3. Has the candidate *demonstrated ascertainment of key public health facts from the material provided* and used it appropriately?

> Bronchioloalveolar carcinoma (BAC) is a type of non-small-cell lung cancer (NSCLC). It makes up 5% of all lung cancers. BAC is more common in women and people who have never smoked. The patient belongs to this subgroup. All candidates must identify this to pass. Good candidates will be able to indicate how many 5% of cases represent in a chosen area, region or national pattern.
>
> Erlotinib is licensed for patients with NSCLC, in whom at least one prior chemotherapy regimen has failed, but guidance does not recommend its use beyond second-line treatment. The patient appears to have had a good response to their self-funded erlotinib and has had no disease progression for more than 1 year.

4. Has the candidate given a *balanced view* and/or *explained appropriately key public health concepts* in a public health setting?

> The candidate should understand that funding is limited and there is an opportunity cost involved in funding decisions. If all applications for individual funding of all new or experimental treatments or those not yet adopted for funding by the healthcare system were approved, as a matter of course, this could result in funding running out before the end of the year. Funding would then just be available on a first come, first served basis. All candidates should identify that there is a limit to healthcare resourcing, hence explaining the processes described here.

5. Has the candidate demonstrated sensitivity in handling *uncertainty, the unexpected, conflict* and/or *responding to challenging questions?*

> The candidate should recognise that Mrs Smith could be considered exceptional, even though she fits into a recognised subgroup and the oncologist did not make a strong case for exceptionality, as her disease has remained stable for more than a year. The candidate should have a view on what should happen next, e.g. suggest discussion with the specialist medicines group chair to review the application if she could be considered exceptional. Failing to identify this possibility or simply defending the current decision would indicate a poor performance. Good candidates should point out that a negative National Institute for Health and Care Excellence (NICE) decision often indicates evidence of relatively poor effectiveness.

Role player briefing pack

ROLE PLAYER BRIEF

You are the director of public health. You have received a phone call from the hospital patient advisory service* (PALS) a short while ago to tell you about a patient with lung cancer, Mrs Smith, who was seen earlier in the day at the oncology clinic. Mrs Smith and her family are threatening to go to the media. Mrs Smith has just found out that a request from her oncologist for funding for erlotinib has been turned down by your healthcare organisation. There has been a lot of media interest recently about funding decisions in relation to anti-cancer drugs.

Decisions about requests for funding high-cost drugs are taken by the organisation's specialist medicines group. You are not a member of that group but one of your public health consultants is, and they have left a briefing for the trainee in anticipation of a possible challenge to the initial decision. As the consultant is on leave, you have therefore asked the trainee to come and speak to you.

You begin by saying:

Tell me about this application to fund erlotinib for Mrs Smith.

You might want to use some prompts such as:

What are the indications and guidance for using erlotinib?

What about any particular indications to treat this patient?

What were the reasons for rejecting the application?

When you have been provided with the briefing you say:

Thank you. We have heard from the hospital that Mrs Smith attended the clinic today and was told that the application for erlotinib funding has been rejected. She and her family are very annoyed about this and are threatening to go to the media.

Wait for any response. Depending on it, add:

There has been a lot of media interest in exceptional funding requests recently. How could we justify this decision to the public?

Then at the 1-minute bell if not before, ask:

So what do you think we should do next?

ANY 'NO GO' AREAS

Any discussion about the pathology or treatment of lung cancer beyond what is provided in the scenario. Any discussion about the issue of co-payments. Any discussion about the pharmacology of erlotinib.

LEVEL OF CONFLICT

Low to moderate. You want to understand the position before deciding on what to do about it.

* A **patient advisory and liaison service** (PALS) is a local NHS service to assist patients with queries about NHS services and care, including signposting for concerns and complaints. It is mainly staffed by experienced NHS employees – usually non-clinicians.

Blank Part B scenario feedback form

SCENARIO 5: EXCEPTIONAL FUNDING REQUEST

ACCESS AT http://goo.gl/ICTj3M

General performance

What was good?
What could be improved?

1. Presenting communication A B C D E

What was good?
What could be improved?

2. Listening and comprehending A B C D E

What was good?
What could be improved?

3. Assimilating relevant information A B C D E

What was good?
What could be improved?

4. Reasoning, analytical and judgement A B C D E

What was good?
What could be improved?

5. Uncertainty and conflict A B C D E

What was good?
What could be improved?

Faculty of Public Health

Of the Royal Colleges of Physicians of the United Kingdom

Working to improve the public's health

Scenario 6

Breast screening uptake rates

(original author Daniel Seddon, edited by Chris Packham and Jill Meara)

Candidate pack

CANDIDATE TASK

You are a member of the public health team which has been asked to advise both on how breast screening rates can be improved locally and how inequalities in rates between different local groups lessened. You are to brief a senior health service manager who is responsible for ensuring the service performs well.

You have 8 minutes to prepare for the station. You are not required to prepare any visual aids. You will then spend 2–3 minutes giving a verbal presentation, and there will then be a discussion for the remainder of the 8 minutes. You may use paper notes.

OUTLINE OF SITUATION

According to the International Agency for Research on Cancer, breast cancer screening reduces mortality by 35% in women who are regularly screened. A breast cancer screening programme is established in your country. The programme aims to detect early cancers in women aged 50–69 years using X ray mammography.

The programme offers screening, once every 3 years, to women who are registered with a general practitioner (GP).* The programme has now completed six rounds of screening (i.e. has been running for around 18 years). A target of 70% coverage, at the health district level, is set by the government.

Performance data for screening rounds 5 and 6 is available (Table 6.3 and Figure 6.1). Using the data for your health district, which comprises 35 GP practices, you have been asked to advise your senior manager on what actions could be taken specifically to improve uptake and, more generally, to lessen inequalities between groups.

CANDIDATE GUIDANCE

Describe what the data shows and how uptake might be improved and inequality reduced.

AT THE STATION

You will be greeted by a marker examiner who will take your candidate number and then hand you over to the role player by saying :

> This is the senior health service manager. They will now start the station.

* A general practitioner is equivalent to a family physician, offering general medical care to a defined population. Usually operates from a community office with no direct hospital beds.

Table 6.3 Round 6 breast screening performance report: 2005–2007

General practice number	Round 5 uptake (%)	Round 6 uptake (%)	Round 6 additional number required to meet target[a]	Number of non-attendees in round 6
1	64	57	38	123
2	66	73	–21	191
3	68	58	43	150
4	60	61	27	115
5	70	70	0	324
6	71	66	17	137
7	72	71	–9	262
8	72	77	–24	79
9	72	72	–17	247
10	72	68	7	97
11	64	73	–26	237
12	74	74	–33	218
13	75	78	–50	138
14	75	75	–47	238
15	75	70	0	164
16	75	75	–20	103
17	76	65	10	69
18	76	75	–72	361
19	76	75	–89	446
20	77	72	–28	393
21	77	74	–18	122
22	77	74	–44	292
23	70	72	–8	116
24	77	74	–7	47
25	78	73	–29	268
26	78	77	–42	139
27	78	80	–54	108
28	78	79	–84	197
29	80	78	–100	275
30	80	79	–30	71
31	80	79	–102	239
32	82	80	–38	76
33	83	82	–90	136
34	83	83	–53	70
35	80	71	–10	317

Source: Screening Information Services.

[a] The target is 70% uptake.

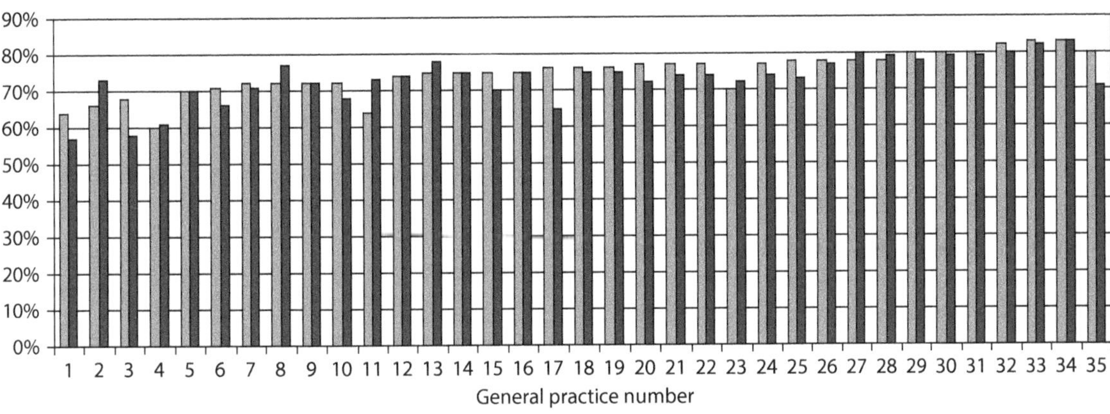

Figure 6.1 Breast screening coverage by practice rounds 5 and 6.

Examiner pack

EXAMINER SITUATION

You will greet the candidate and record their number and name and then hand over to the role player saying:

> This is the senior health service manager. They will now start the station.

EXAMINER ANSWER GUIDANCE

The candidate should be able to identify and communicate the basic statistical and interpretive aspects of this station, as well as to communicate essential elements of screening programmes. However, the station is as much about change management and how information can be communicated to support quality improvement.

FACTS FROM THE INFORMATION GIVEN

- Overall apparent slight decrease in uptake between rounds 5 and 6.
- Only six practices below target in round 6.
- Two practices that were below target in round 5 were at or above target in round 6.
- Practice size (number of patients invited) can be calculated from the data given, though candidates are not expected to do this. A good candidate would indicate that they would want to analyse whether there was correlation between practice size and uptake rates, and indicate possible methods.

FACTORS THAT MAY ALTER UPTAKE RATES

Candidates should offer:

- Socioeconomic factors.
- Ethnicity.
- Age structure of the practice (not a strong factor as the screening is only for a 20-year age band and only rarely would practice populations differ significantly between such age bands).
- Attitude of the primary care team to the programme as evidenced by, e.g. availability of literature in the waiting room, opportunistic encouragement to attend.
- Ease of getting to the screening location (many areas have mobile facilities that may be sited in one practice car park to cover a number of practices). Other patients may need to travel to a hospital for screening.
- Link between uptake and a possible reflection of inequalities in other health areas.

STRATEGIES TO WORK WITH PRIMARY CARE TEAMS TO IMPROVE UPTAKE

- Provide feedback of data to practices, anonymised but with each practice shown their own position.
- Focus on practices below target or where performance has decreased by more than a couple of percentage points between screening rounds.
- Ask the high-performing practices if they have specific strategies that improve performance, and then share these with all practices.
- Discuss the role of financial or other incentives in improving uptake rates.

EFFECTS OF IMPROVING UPTAKE ON PUBLIC HEALTH

- Despite a target of 70% there would be greater health benefit if higher uptake rates were achieved.
- An excellent candidate would use their background knowledge of the breast screening programme to estimate that if the roughly 140 extra screened patients needed to meet the target in the below target practices were screened, it is likely that one additional cancer would be detected, but a number of women would be called back for further tests.

EXAMINER BRIEFING PACK

Marking guide for examiners

1. Has the candidate appropriately demonstrated *presenting skills* in a typical public health setting (presenting to a person or audience)?

> Summarises clearly, with emphasis on key points. Avoids jargon. Uses eye contact and non-verbal communication. Able to extract key points from data and to ignore extraneous detail.

2. Has the candidate appropriately demonstrated *listening skills* in a typical public health setting (listening and responding appropriately)?

> Invites questions, pauses and listens. Understands questions and responds appropriately including seeking clarification.

3. Has the candidate *demonstrated ascertainment of key public health facts from the material provided* and used it appropriately?

> The table shows practice-by-practice variation, with some practices improving and some worsening between rounds. The candidate should propose possible reasons for these differences such as ethnic, socio-demographic and access differences between practices to pass.
>
> A good candidate will realise that practice sizes can be deduced from the number needed to meet target. A good candidate will comment that they would want to analyse whether there was any correlation between practice size and uptake rates and say how they might do this.
>
> Candidates should appreciate that small differences in uptake between rounds are unlikely to be clinically or statistically significant. Excessive focus on those indicates a weak performance.

4. Has the candidate given a *balanced view* and/or *explained appropriately key public health concepts* in a public health setting?

> Possible reasons for variations in performance should be linked with other preventive aspects of general practice such as other screening programmes, immunisation programmes and case findings.
>
> A good candidate will quickly focus on those practices that perform particularly well or particularly badly, especially where there is a large change between rounds. They will see opportunities for learning from good practice and for supporting underperformers.
>
> To pass, all candidates should mention opportunities for communication and feedback to practices: good candidates will suggest ranking the chart. Candidates should realise that it may not be appropriate to show named data from all the practices to each individual practices; anonymisation may be needed.

5. Has the candidate demonstrated sensitivity in handling *uncertainty, the unexpected, conflict* and/or *responding to challenging questions?*

> A good candidate will discuss the role of financial or other incentives or penalties in improving uptake rates and discuss how to influence general practitioners when their pay may not be affected by this area of performance.
>
> An excellent candidate would use their background knowledge of the breast screening programme to estimate that if the roughly 140 extra screened patients needed to meet the target in the below-target practices were screened, it is likely that one additional cancer would be detected, but a number of women would be called back for further tests.

Role player briefing pack

STATION BACKGROUND

As candidate briefing.

ROLE PLAYER BRIEF

You want to see improved screening coverage so that fewer people die of cancer. You are aware that in the case of breast cancer screening, GPs are not paid directly for enhancing screening coverage in their populations.

You want to understand the present performance and hear a convincing case made for how GPs can be persuaded to take a stronger interest in their own population coverage. You consider a target of 70% coverage for a life-saving screening test to be much too low. You are used to targets of 100% compliance with standards.

Candidate will give 2- to 3-minute verbal presentation, after which you should ask the following questions, if not adequately covered in the presentation.

Start by asking:

Some rates are falling. I detect a difference between screening rounds. What might lie behind this?

Follow up with:

What lies behind the differences in performance between practices?

Do you think it's the smaller single-handed practices that are not doing so well?

[Candidate should indicate possible analysis to correlate practice size and uptake rates.]

If we want to improve uptake rates, what do you suggest we do? Which practices should we be focusing on?

How do you suggest we encourage the poorer-performing practices?

Surely we should be aiming for better than 70% uptake. How much will improving our screening coverage make a difference to people's health?

ANY 'NO GO' AREAS

None.

LEVEL OF CONFLICT

Medium. The candidate should acknowledge that the practices may be resistant to change and they may not feel that a 70% uptake rate is too bad.

Blank Part B scenario feedback form

SCENARIO 6: BREAST SCREENING UPTAKE RATES

ACCESS AT Access at http://goo.gl/ANM1pH

General performance

What was good?
What could be improved?

1. **Presenting communication** A B C D E

What was good?
What could be improved?

2. **Listening and comprehending** A B C D E

What was good?
What could be improved?

3. **Assimilating relevant information** A B C D E

What was good?
What could be improved?

4. **Reasoning, analytical and judgement** A B C D E

What was good?
What could be improved?

5. **Uncertainty and conflict** A B C D E

What was good?
What could be improved?

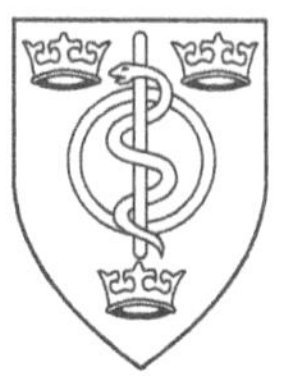

Faculty of Public Health

Of the Royal Colleges of Physicians of the United Kingdom

Working to improve the public's health

Scenario 7

Emergency hospital admissions

(original author Bruce Bolam, edited by Chris Packham and Jill Meara)

Candidate pack

CANDIDATE TASK

You are a member of a public health team in your health organisation.* Your chief executive wishes to discuss data with you that he or she has seen that evaluates if work by an 'older people's task group' to reduce emergency hospital admissions from care homes has been successful.

You have 8 minutes to prepare for the station. You are not required to prepare any visual aids. At the station you will spend 2–3 minutes giving a verbal presentation, and there will then be a discussion with the role player. You may use paper notes to aid your verbal briefing. The station will last a total of 8 minutes.

OUTLINE OF SITUATION

Your organisation is responsible for a population of 200,000, which is relatively affluent and elderly. A sustained project (older people's task group) to try and reduce emergency admissions to hospital has been underway for the last 3 years. This focused on improving the quality of clinical and social care in care homes (residential, nursing and other care homes†). You have only a brief description of the work (in the candidate pack). However, you have discussed this with the task group leader and know that reports to date have shown significant improvements in the quality of clinical care in some of these homes, with improvements in care home residents' satisfaction surveys and a reduction in untoward incidents and reported prescribing errors.

A recent analysis of emergency admissions among older people has been carried out by one of the analysts in your team (also in the candidate briefing pack). The chief executive of your organisation has seen the data and wishes to meet with you to discuss.

CANDIDATE GUIDANCE

Describe the key findings from the data and consider the implications for planning future interventions to reduce emergency admissions.

AT THE STATION

You will be greeted by a marker examiner who will take your candidate number and name and then hand over to the role player by saying:

> This is the chief executive. They will now start the station.

* A **primary care organisation** (PCO) is an NHS organisation that provides community and primary healthcare and commissions healthcare from community and hospital services. In England these are called primary care trusts (PCTs). A health board in Scotland performs some similar functions. PCTs and health boards generally cover designated areas and populations within those areas.

† 'Care homes' refers to any form of institutional care provided privately or by a local authority (council) to care for mainly elderly residents who are too frail to manage independently in their own homes. In this scenario this includes residential homes, care homes, nursing homes and sheltered accommodation, which are all considered to be different varieties of care homes.

CANDIDATE BRIEFING PACK

Item 1

Brief description of the older people's task group work

The group were set up in 2006 to try and tackle what were perceived as high levels of inappropriate emergency hospital admissions from residential care homes. The group comprised managers and clinicians from primary and secondary care that covered the district (population approximately 200,000) and the main hospital receiving emergency admissions. The group identified a range of interventions and these were put in place, including more intensive prescribed medicine reviews, strengthened primary care activity within certain residential homes and more formal incident reporting agreed upon by residential and nursing home managers.

Item 2 (Tables 6.4 and 6.5)

Table 6.4 Crude age-specific (aged 65 and over) rate of emergency admissions per 1000 persons, with 95% confidence intervals, by home type and area of residence for 2005–2006

Area and type of residence	Population size[a]	Total emergency admissions[a]	Rate per 1000	Lower 95% CI	Upper 95% CI
All care homes	4456	1337	300	284	317
Nursing homes	1017	285	280	250	315
Residential homes	930	357	384	346	426
Sheltered accommodation	1816	465	256	234	280
All non-care home sources	32,241	5411	168	163	172
All sources (whole population)	36,697	6748	184	180	188
Regional average	164,233	33,733	205	203	208

[a] Aged 65 and over.

Table 6.5 Relative percentage change in the crude age-specific (aged 65 and older) rate of emergency admissions by home type and area of residence for 2 successive year periods

	Relative % change for 2 successive year periods	
Area and type of residence	2005–2006[a] to 2006–2007[a]	2006–2007[a] to 2007–2008[a]
All care homes	+19	+15
Nursing homes	+26	+11
Residential homes	+22	+18
Sheltered accommodation	+9	+14
All non-care home sources	+7	+4
All sources (whole population)	+9	+7
Regional average	+5	+6

[a] 2005/2006 and subsequent year data refers to financial years (April 2005–March 2006) not to calendar years.

Examiner pack

EXAMINER SITUATION

You will greet the candidate and record their candidate number and name and then hand over to the role player by saying:

> This is the chief executive. They will now start the station.

EXAMINER ANSWER GUIDANCE

The station requires the candidate to describe some basic activity data and identify that which is robust and that which requires more information (such as time trends) before sensible conclusions can be drawn. The immediate question targets the worth of the older people's task group work. Good candidates should identify a wider concern about whether any work is required in the non-residential home population.

The candidate should identify from the chief executive's questions that uncertainty exists in his or her mind as to the effectiveness of the initiative – which is not described in detail but which has been running for 3 years. Weak candidates will fail to describe possible reasons for the apparent failure: audit about what has actually been implemented, lack of size, not enough people being affected by an intervention, lack of evidence that the intervention works (although the information presented shows some measures that appear to have been positively affected), lack of time to take effect and lack of statistically significant trends.

EXAMINER BRIEFING PACK

Marking guide for examiners

Specific marking guidance is carefully prepared to indicate to you when a candidate should fail (or excel) at a particular competency based on core material from the scenario. However, we recognise that we cannot anticipate all possible candidate responses. If a candidate says something that in your view merits a Grade E (or indicates excellence – Grade A) on that competency or station that we have not explicitly included in the marking guidance, it is important that you do then mark the candidate as a fail (or indicate excellence). In that situation, you need to operate outside the specific marking guidance, but please detail the issue in the examination feedback.

1. Has the candidate appropriately demonstrated *presenting skills* in a typical public health setting (presenting to a person or audience)?

Avoids jargon. Is clear. Appropriate language for the audience. Maintains eye contact. Appropriate manner for the situation. Shows empathy.

2. Has the candidate appropriately demonstrated *listening skills* in a typical public health setting (listening and responding appropriately)?

Ensures role player questions are answered appropriately. Answers totality of the question. Manner of response appropriate to role player scenario.

3. Has the candidate *demonstrated ascertainment of key public health facts from the material provided* and used it appropriately?

To pass, candidates should describe:

- Data quality: Importance of ensuring 95% CIs and trends over time are statistically robust. Data does not allow conclusions about subsequent year's trends.
- Relative percentage change in the crude age-specific (aged 65 and older) rate of emergency admissions for 2 successive year periods, i.e. remains positive.
- Variations in admission rates from different types of homes and the wider community; baseline data shows significantly higher admission rates from residential homes than other types of homes, or from non-home sources. The absolute numbers of admissions, with a minority from residential homes and nursing homes (least).

4. Has the candidate given a *balanced view* and/or *explained appropriately key public health concepts* in a public health setting?

All candidates should acknowledge the lack of strong evidence for the impact of the older people's task group to perform adequately, while highlighting the need for longer-term trend data; the impact of the work of the older people's task group may take some time to show an effect – mention the lower percentage increase in the 2006–2007 to 2007–2008 year (most recent) – lack of statistical analysis makes interpretation difficult. Good candidates may identify that the overall area rate is significantly lower than the regional average so that new significant reductions may not be expected or appropriate.

To pass this section, candidates should be able to comment on the fact that possible proxy indicators that reflect quality (such as reduced prescribing errors) may be important.

5. Has the candidate demonstrated sensitivity in handling *uncertainty, the unexpected, conflict* and/or *responding to challenging questions?*

The candidate should respond appropriately to the question concerning why the work of the task group to improve the quality of care in local care homes isn't necessarily reflected in the data. Responds objectively to questions on the focus on older people.

Candidates should respond to the suggestion it is simply due to more frail elderly with appropriate caution. Discuss possible need to look at non-care home population despite lower than regional admission rates.

Role player briefing pack

STATION BACKGROUND

As candidate briefing.

ROLE PLAYER BRIEF

You are playing the part of the chief executive of the local primary care organisation (PCO). You were involved in supporting the work on reducing emergency hospital admissions by suggesting care homes may be a fruitful place to start. This followed a visit you made some 4 years ago to the local hospital where one of the medical consultants showed you two patients who had been admitted from a care home due to the side effects from 'cocktails' of prescribed drugs. At the same time, your elderly mother died following a fall in another care home many miles away. These events focused your thoughts on improving care in such institutions. You have supported the older people's task group initiative focusing on care homes, and you firmly believe in the value of the work. However, you feel that the presented results do not reflect well on the impact of the task group.

Start the station by saying:

Please very briefly summarise the findings.

What do you think these findings tell us about reducing emergency admissions among older people in our patch?

How could the data be improved?

Then:

Is it true that these results show the older people's team hasn't been effective in reducing emergency admissions from care homes?

[Candidates should give a coherent answer either way – if they don't mention a delay in effect not yet translated into annual activity, prompt them – this indicates a weaker performance.]

And then:

Well could it be due to more and more frail people going into these homes?

[Candidates should not accept this: random variation, alternatively admission or on-call arrangements, new or recently closed alternative facilities, changes in staffing or patient pathway practices.]

And:

How could we investigate that?

The candidate does not necessarily expect you to ask about improvements in the quality of care in care homes. You should ask them:

What do you think about the task group's work to improve the quality of care in local care homes?

[Weak candidates will fail to link the reported quality markers as possible proxies of effective interventions, especially following the scripted prompting.]

Then:

So what is your advice about what we should be doing now?

If the candidate hasn't mentioned it at all, ask:

Should we be looking at the non-care homes population?

[Candidate should be able to suggest a way forward, including specifying what sort of information they would seek to help provide additional assessment of the initiative. The scenario is purposefully vague to test out candidates' ability to propose more detailed actions and evaluation.]

ANY 'NO GO' AREAS

None.

LEVEL OF CONFLICT

Medium.

Blank Part B scenario feedback form

SCENARIO 7: EMERGENCY HOSPITAL ADMISSIONS

ACCESS AT http://goo.gl/Lgka1m

General performance

What was good?
What could be improved?

1. Presenting communication A B C D E

What was good?
What could be improved?

2. Listening and comprehending A B C D E

What was good?
What could be improved?

3. Assimilating relevant information A B C D E

What was good?
What could be improved?

4. Reasoning, analytical and judgement A B C D E

What was good?
What could be improved?

5. Uncertainty and conflict A B C D E

What was good?
What could be improved?

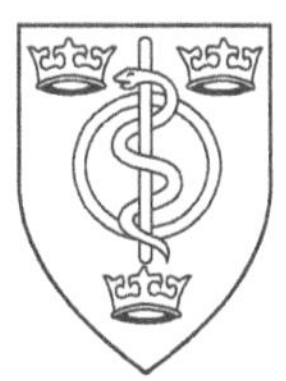

Faculty of Public Health

Of the Royal Colleges of Physicians of the United Kingdom

Working to improve the public's health

Scenario 8

Smoking ban

(original author Christine Hine, edited by Chris Packham and Jill Meara)

Candidate pack

CANDIDATE TASK

You work in a local health service public health team. You are to speak over the **telephone** to a local newspaper journalist who is about to ring you. The journalist would like to hear your response to claims that a national ban on smoking in public places, introduced some 2 years earlier, is not working.

You have 8 minutes to prepare for the station. You will then spend 8 minutes discussing the task with a role player. You may use paper notes to aid your verbal briefing.

OUTLINE OF SITUATION

The local journalist recently interviewed the owner of three local bars. The bar owner claimed that research from your department shows that the ban has not had any useful impact on people smoking. Businesses like his are losing customers because the smoking ban has reduced their enjoyment of a visit to a local bar. He believes the ban should be lifted immediately. The journalist would like to hear your response.

CANDIDATE GUIDANCE

You have a summary of results from a before and after study of smoking prevalence and weekly cigarette consumption in a local population sample. The surveys were conducted by the public health department that you work in and have been published in the latest annual report of the director of public health (DPH). You also have a summary of findings of a different research study into second-hand smoke exposure of workers in the hospitality industry. This was conducted elsewhere in the county but over a similar time period (both studies summarised in the candidate pack). The journalist already has the same briefing material.

You should prepare to explain the findings of the two studies and respond to the journalist's questions.

AT THE STATION

You will be greeted by a marker examiner who will take your candidate number and name and then you will be told:

> Please sit down and wait for the telephone call from the journalist. This will start the station.

CANDIDATE BRIEFING PACK

1. **Summary of local before and after study of smoking**

   Questionnaires were sent to a random sample of people registered with general practices in your health district prior to the introduction of a national ban on smoking in enclosed public spaces. The postal survey was repeated with a second random sample 3 months after the ban was implemented. The sample size was 4000 and returns of 2350 (59%) were expected, sufficient to detect a decline in smoking of 3.5% with 80% power at the 0.5% significance level.

   The response rates were 61% and 57%, respectively. There were no significant differences in the age, gender and ethnicity profile of the respondents. Data completeness was satisfactory in both surveys. Smoking status was established in 96% of questionnaires for each survey. Results are provided in Table 6.6.

The standardised prevalence of smoking adjusted to the age and gender profile of your health district was 22.5% before the ban and 22.7% afterwards – this was not a statistically significant difference.

The proportion of smokers reporting average consumption of 20 or more cigarettes daily fell following the ban (Table 6.7). One-tailed Fisher's exact test for proportion of current smokers smoking in excess of 20 a day across the two surveys had a p value of 0.0439, statistically significant at the 0.05 level.

2. **Changes in second-hand smoke exposure in hospitality sector businesses following introduction of a ban on smoking in enclosed public spaces**

Salivary cotinine levels were measured in 80 non-smoking employees of 50 businesses 1 month before and 1 month after the introduction of the ban. Members of a smoking cessation team invited bars and restaurants on their mailing list to participate. Two non-smoking employees at each business were invited to provide saliva samples. Only employees not exposed to any other source of smoke (e.g. smokers at home) were included. Anyone smoking within the past year was excluded.

Results were analysed for all 80 employees (the cross-sectional group) and for 42 employees from 30 businesses for whom matched samples were available and hence a matched analysis was possible (Table 6.8). Salivary cotinine levels fell by approximately 75% following the ban.

Table 6.6 Smoking status in the before and after survey samples

Smoking status	Before smoking ban % (95% CI)	3 months after the ban % (95% CI)
Current smokers	21.2 (19.4–23.0)	21.1 (19.2–22.9)
Ex-smokers	37.2 (34.9–39.2)	36.7 (34.4–38.8)
Never smoked	41.9 (39.7–44.0)	42.5 (40.2–44.7)

Total % may not add up to 100% due to rounding.

Table 6.7 Smokers averaging 20 or more daily cigarettes each week

	Number before the smoking ban	% before the smoking ban (95% CI)	Number 3 months after the smoking ban	% 3 months after the smoking ban (95% CI)
Current smokers reporting number of cigarettes smoked	370	–	353	–
Number averaging 20 or more cigarettes smoked daily	102	27.6 (23.3–32.3)	77	21.8* (17.7–26.6)

*$p = 0.0439$, statistically significant at the 0.05 level.

Table 6.8 Salivary continine levels before and after the introduction of the ban

	Baseline salivary cotinine level	Post-ban salivary cotinine level
Cross-sectional analysis ($n = 75$)	3.5 ng/mL	0.9 ng/mL*
Matched analysis ($n = 39$)	3.7 ng/mL	1.0 ng/mL*

*$p < 0.001$.

Examiner pack

EXAMINER SITUATION

The marker examiner will take the candidate number and name, and then the candidate will be told:

> Please sit down and wait for the telephone call from the journalist. This will start the station.

EXAMINER ANSWER GUIDANCE

This OSPHE gives candidates the opportunity to show how they can respond sensitively to problems for those adversely affected by measures to improve health, while communicating clear public health messages in support of a smoking ban and early evidence of benefits (notably among workers who had previously been exposed to smoke in their workplace).

In discussing evidence, they should draw on both studies summarised in their briefing pack. It is very important that the candidate's answer includes the need to reduce passive smoking among occupationally exposed workers (and possible early indications of success in achieving this).

EXAMINER BRIEFING PACK

Marking guide for examiners

Specific marking guidance is carefully prepared to indicate to you when a candidate should fail (or excel) at a particular competency based on core material from the scenario. However, we recognise that we cannot anticipate all possible candidate responses. If a candidate says something that in your view merits a fail (or indicates excellence) on that competency or station that we have not explicitly included in the marking guidance, it is important that you then mark the candidate as a fail (or indicate excellence). In that situation, you need to operate outside the specific marking guidance, but please detail the issue in the examination feedback.

1. Has the candidate appropriately demonstrated *presenting skills* in a typical public health setting (presenting to a person or audience)?

> Avoids jargon. Is clear. Appropriate language for the audience. Appropriate manner for the situation. Shows empathy.

2. Has the candidate appropriately demonstrated *listening skills* in a typical public health setting (listening and responding appropriately)?

> Ensures role player questions are answered appropriately. Answers totality of the question. Manner of response appropriate to role player scenario.

3. Has the candidate *demonstrated ascertainment of key public health facts from the material provided* and used it appropriately?

> The candidate must clearly identify the following to pass:
>
> Smoking prevalence did not change when reassessed 3 months after the introduction of a ban on smoking in enclosed public spaces
>
> There was a statistically significant fall in smokers reporting an average daily consumption of 20 or more cigarettes.
>
> For the first local study, data issues about the proportion of the respondents who gave a smoking history that included numbers of cigarettes smoked in both questionnaires (370 out of approximately 2300) are important, as there may be significant selection bias in this. Good candidates will handle this carefully – acknowledging this possible bias without losing the positive message from the observed effect in those 370 persons.

All candidates must describe the study results showing a fall in salivary cotinine levels among hospitality sector employees 1 month after the introduction of the ban.

4. Has the candidate given a *balanced view* and/or *explained appropriately key public health concepts* in a public health setting?

Candidates must acknowledge the methodological limitations of the before and after population survey (e.g. self-reported smoking status) and timing (possibility of reassessing prevalence too soon after the ban) to perform averagely. Findings on early benefits to occupationally exposed workers are very important: reducing passive smoking is a prime benefit of the smoking ban, and candidates must identify this to pass. Candidates should demonstrate a wide knowledge of the hazards of smoking to support and reinforce the value of the ban, including the problems of second-hand smoke, value of primary prevention, need for programmes rather than single interventions to reduce smoking and need to prevent involuntary exposure of employees.

5. Has the candidate demonstrated sensitivity in handling *uncertainty, the unexpected, conflict* and/or *responding to challenging questions?*

The candidate responds to concerns about negative impacts on businesses sensitively. They may note potential benefits to businesses, e.g. achieving a healthier workforce. They may raise the need to investigate the scale of this problem and what might be done to tackle it without compromising the benefits of the ban. They do not accept that local research is worthless because of a conflict of interest in the public health department: evaluation and monitoring of health impacts is a necessary function. Use of independent rather than in-house researchers may have increased local credibility of the research. They are confident in conveying the public health message that whatever the strengths and weaknesses of local research, there is overwhelming evidence to support continued action to reduce the harm caused by smoking, and the ban is a very important part of this.

Role player briefing pack

STATION BACKGROUND

This station is about justification of a recently introduced ban on smoking in enclosed public spaces. Part of the justification is the need to reduce passive occupational exposure, e.g. among bar and restaurant staff. The candidate has a copy of research (which you are aware of) which they should use to support their arguments in support of the smoking ban.

ROLE PLAYER BRIEF

You are a local newspaper journalist. You recently interviewed the owner of three town centre bars. He feels angry about the ban on smoking in enclosed public spaces. Profit margins have been tight for some years. In the first 6 months since the ban was introduced, one of his bars recorded a 20% fall in profits, and that fall has continued since (although the other two have seen little change). You have never smoked but are interested in arguments about the state interfering with personal lifestyle choices.

You intend to quiz the local public health department and see if they will admit that the ban has not been as successful as hoped. Their department published local research on smoking before and after the ban was introduced which shows no significant change in the numbers of people smoking. You read a short summary of this in the annual report of the local director of public health. There is also a finding about fewer cigarettes being smoked each week, but you feel this is small print. You think the public health department is unlikely to be an objective source of this type of research, as trying to reduce smoking is a major part of their role.

You will ask tough questions but allow the candidate time to put forward their arguments. You will start by saying:

> **Thank you for talking to me and giving me this background information. I understand that you have to say that smoking is not good for people, but as research from your own department shows that the ban is not succeeding, isn't it time to say that this ban should be lifted? It's harming local businesses!**
>
> **You found that some people might be smoking fewer cigarettes, but some of the business people that I've interviewed are not convinced! Surely people completing your questionnaires can just lie about how much they smoke?**
>
> **What's wrong with people enjoying a cigarette when they visit a bar or restaurant?**
>
> **Your small local study does not seem a very substantial body of evidence!**
>
> **A local bar owner has told me that they always used to have no-smoking areas for customers who don't like smoke. They were very successful. He can't understand why he can't carry on providing these smoke-free areas rather than spoiling everyone else's enjoyment of a night out.**
>
> **We've previously featured local services that help people who want to stop smoking to actually give up. Wouldn't it be better for your department to concentrate on providing more of these rather than interfering with how people choose to enjoy themselves in their spare time?**

At the 1-minute bell (unless already clearly covered):

> **Finally, why should local business owners go along with supporting this ban, even though it is harming them?**

ANY 'NO GO' AREAS

None.

LEVEL OF CONFLICT

Medium level of conflict.

Blank Part B scenario feedback form

SCENARIO 8: SMOKING BAN

ACCESS AT http://goo.gl/Gbn7Iz

General performance

What was good?
What could be improved?

1. **Presenting communication** A B C D E

What was good?
What could be improved?

2. **Listening and comprehending** A B C D E

What was good?
What could be improved?

3. **Assimilating relevant information** A B C D E

What was good?
What could be improved?

4. **Reasoning, analytical and judgement** A B C D E

What was good?
What could be improved?

5. **Uncertainty and conflict** A B C D E

What was good?
What could be improved?

PART B SCENARIO FEEDBACK FORMS COMPLETED BY A TEAM OF EXPERIENCED MARKERS*

Scenario 1: Infection hazards of human cadavers

General performance

What was good? Confident, clear, calm, reassuring performance.
What could be improved? Checking understanding and that all concerns had been addressed.
Key tip for candidate: check understanding to ensure the role player is following you.

1. **Presenting communication** (A) B C D E

What was good? Candidate introduced herself well. Clear and reassuring. Sympathetic without being patronising. Good empathy. Good eye contact. No jargon. No inappropriate overtechnical language used. Empathetic. Answers were clear and not too long.
What could be improved? Candidate tended to be very positive – an edge of caution would improve matters.

2. **Listening and comprehending** (A) B C D E

What was good? Answered all questions appropriately having picked up on points being raised. Not dismissive or patronising. Showed was listening to concerns.
What could be improved? Checking that all concerns had been addressed.

* The marks below and comments have been agreed by three past or current OSPHE examiners who are thanked for their time and diligence: Dr Annette Wood, Consultant in Public Health, Public Health England; Dr John Linnane, Director of Public Health, Warwickshire County Council UK; and Dr Rob Cooper, Head of School of Public Health, NHS Health Education England. These marks relate to the standard as used in 2014.

3. Assimilating relevant information A (B) C D E

What was good?
Covered brief without the need for excessive prompts. Covered general issues – such as masks and general precautions – then concentrated on specifics of smallpox and anthrax.
What could be improved?
Not to be inaccurate over history of anthrax infection. Said 'no cases of anthrax in past 200 years', which is not entirely true. Could have discussed more issues around open/closed working conditions and lack of evidence of historical transmission to workers and risks to workers of using lime.

4. Reasoning, analytical and judgement (A) B C D E

What was good?
Covered risks from wood, spores and lead rather than focusing on anthrax or smallpox.
What could be improved?
Covered general aspects of brief but risks were maybe not put into the context of other risks, so could have given more advice on reducing the health risks to workforce, e.g. ensuring robust ongoing health and safety at work training in place. Said not to use lime and then said other things could be used to disinfect the site; this gives a confusing message – either the site needs to be disinfected or it does not.

5. Uncertainty and conflict (A) B C D E

What was good?
Appreciated concerns. Very good summary. Responded to risk issues (e.g. coffins and plague pit) and pay as outlined in brief and did not consider situation beyond what would have been the responsibility of public health. Agreed with national health and safety regulator.
What could be improved?
Could have given an overview of experts who could be involved, e.g. chemical and biological expertise from recognised national sources. Be careful not to acknowledge risks beyond that which she is qualified to talk about which might make job risky, i.e. construction in an urban area, but was clear it is nothing to do with her, e.g. mentioned 'other more modern methods available', but this information was not in the briefing material.

Scenario 2: Land contamination in a residential area

General performance

What was good?
Good confident clear introduction, showed empathy, reassuring, helpful and proactive about offering advice/solutions to problems.
What could be improved?
Check understanding, some answers were a little long, often referred to notes.
Key tip for candidate: make sure you are always answering the question asked. If you think the question is unreasonable, you still need to acknowledge it and explain why it is not relevant/suitable, etc. before moving forward.

1. **Presenting communication** A (B) C D E

What was good?
Candidate introduced himself well. Gave clear introduction. Reassuring. Showed empathy. Addressed most issues. No jargon.
What could be improved?
Could have used less technical language or else explained technical terms/processes and made answers a bit shorter as was at the end, pushed for time. Could have checked understanding with audience.

2. **Listening and comprehending** A (B) C D E

What was good?
Did respond to questions and concerns, i.e. 'continue to monitor'. Empathy OK.
What could be improved?
Initial response sounded like not dealing with the issue. Sounded dismissive throughout – 'have to have industrial development somewhere' (tough). Avoid saying, 'This is an emotive topic'. Perhaps came across with a lack of sincerity. Didn't really answer the question 'why weren't we told sooner?'

3. Assimilating relevant information A (B) C D E

What was good?
Had understanding of key technical issues. Population health overall covered satisfactorily. Did outline relative health of local area to national area very clearly. Clear about chemicals/side effects. Good example of variation possible street by street.
What could be improved?
Approach to monitoring appeared dismissive and not presented or explained as well as it could have been. Did not necessarily talk about downstream effects, occupational/environmental and lack of evidence as proof that there is no risk.

4. Reasoning, analytical and judgement A (B) C D E

What was good?
Did talk about 'healthy living', i.e. lifestyle issues. Covered short-term issues of carbon disulphate.
What could be improved?
Didn't set in context of wider risks of day-to-day life, i.e. smoking/pollution. It came across with perhaps some victim blaming.

5. Uncertainty and conflict A (B) C D E

What was good?
Didn't duck issues. Offered to come to meeting to speak to local residents and to pass on to colleague house price concerns. Offered to guarantee continued monitoring of local disease rates.
What could be improved?
Language could be more supportive. Could have best avoided any comments himself on house price concerns. A bit hesitant/unsure over whether safe to live near.

Scenario 3: HPV vaccine to prevent cervical cancer

General performance

What was good?
Not much apart from stance and body language were OK.
What could be improved?
Not to provide too detailed answers – make the most of the opportunity to shine. Do not just repeat previous answers as: • This will not get you more marks. • It is frustrating for the role player and sounds rude/dismissive/condescending. • If the GP is asking you a new question, it is because they want you to cover a new area of the scenario so try to provide the information requested.
Key tip for candidate: make the most of the opportunity. Treat each scenario as an 8-minute job interview, and if you find yourself just repeating answers to earlier questions, you need to think about what extra element of the scenario the role player is trying to get you to speak about and then address this area.

1. **Presenting communication** A B C D (E)

What was good?
Not much apart from stance and body language OK.
What could be improved?
Very abrupt. Rather quiet and unconfident. Answer finished after about 4½ minutes. Too much jargon. Don't use abbreviations. Expand on answers. Talk at more appropriate level.

2. **Listening and comprehending** A B C (D) E

What was good?
Very little.
What could be improved?
Did not answer all the questions. Used abbreviations without explanations such as JCVI. Some of the questions either were not answered in totality (one reason why the scenario only lasted 4½ minutes) or the answer was to a different question (repeating earlier question). No recognition of the pressure the GP might be under.

3. Assimilating relevant information A B C (D) E

What was good?
Explained efficacy.
What could be improved?
Limited summary of situation. Repeatedly referred to efficacy without further explanation. More balanced explanation of key facts needed from brief.

4. Reasoning, analytical and judgement A B C D (E)

What was good?
Very little.
What could be improved?
Unbalanced answer which did not cover many areas. More information/discussion on access, how long the screening programme might be in place for, how to manage the media, etc.

5. Uncertainty and conflict A B C (D) E

What was good?
Very little.
What could be improved?
Unbalanced answer which did not cover many areas. Saying it was good – but not recommended and not cost effective. Wider discussion as outlined above, e.g. potential increase in risk-taking behaviour not covered.

Scenario 4: Interview on speed cameras

General performance

What was good? Use of data/evidence to support argument, was not influenced by the interviewer, confident clear start.
What could be improved? The candidate had a condescending, dismissive attitude to the reporter that would only encourage a negative article to be written in the paper.
Key tip for candidate: the exam is not simply an oral exam where you need to state an evidence-based public health position; it is also testing the 'art' of public health. Treating the scenario less like an exam and more like a real-life situation may result in a more empathetic approach. Considering the role players' role and who they are supposed to be representing may also help.

1. **Presenting communication** A B C (D) E

What was good? Introduced himself. Maintained eye contact.
What could be improved? Change in attitude and approach. Poorly presented. Patronising in attitude. Mumbled in places.

2. **Listening and comprehending** A B C (D) E

What was good? Brief and succinct.
What could be improved? Needs to listen and respond to audience. Generally dismissive of audience. Talked over them.

3. Assimilating relevant information A B C (D) E

What was good? Calm responses. Not agitated by reporter.
What could be improved? Unbalanced perspective. Too positive. Limited detail provided in response to questions. Acknowledge limitations.

4. Reasoning, analytical and judgement A B C (D) E

What was good? Very little.
What could be improved? Give balance view of all data provided. Explanation of how cameras are placed to refute some points. Wider explanation of road safety. Only talked about speed cameras. Next to nothing about other aspects of road safety.

5. Uncertainty and conflict A B C (D) E

What was good? Very little.
What could be improved? Inadequate summary. Patronising approach to reporter. Summary needs to be more than just speed cameras.

Scenario 5: Exceptional funding request

General performance

What was good? Stated facts clearly. Not hesitant.
What could be improved? Pace interaction better. The scenario was more than 6½ minutes and this was taken up with the role player trying to extract information and the candidate repeating information or not answering questions. Eye contact, empathy, try to be as helpful as possible.
Key tip for candidate: in the 8 minutes try to be as helpful as possible. One of the key strengths of public health is in its power to influence others and these 8 minutes are testing, among other things, how you are likely to be viewed by colleagues. If someone comes to you with a problem, the key success factor is whether they are better positioned to deal with the situation after your intervention. Good body language and a positive, proactive approach are the bare minimums you should be bringing to these scenarios.

1. **Presenting communication** A B C (D) E

What was good? Stated facts clearly. Not hesitant. Appropriate language.
What could be improved? No introduction. Reading verbatim from paper. Scratching/messing with glasses. No eye contact. Fidgety. Unsure about names. Lack of empathy. General fidgeting. Need to be clear/focused/enthusiastic.

2. **Listening and comprehending** A B C D (E)

What was good? Answered some of the questions.
What could be improved? No eye contact/kept reading and fiddling with paper. Not responding to issues raised by DPH, e.g. whether should go to media. Need to be more helpful/less defensive/less defensive/sound less cold. Did not answer all questions. Responses given tended to be brief. Manner a little aloof. Not to evade questions. Answer the totality of the question. Look for non-verbal prompts to ensure latter has happened.

3. Assimilating relevant information A B (C) D E

What was good?
Seemed to understand basic issue but not with any certainty.
What could be improved?
Poorly briefed – dismissive. Appeared poorly prepared so little/no good. Just read from paper. Be clearer about the patient, process, and condition. Outlined details regarding cancer and drug under question. All answers brief. Rarity of condition not really explored. Give more detail. Seek reassurance that audience understands.

4. Reasoning, analytical and judgement A B C (D) E

What was good?
Cancer drugs fund/talked about process/discussed need for fairness. Stated need for more information.
What could be improved?
Appeared disinterested. Could be more helpful. Outlined issue regarding funding all requests but in a very defensive manner. Only useful suggestion was to speak to surgeon. Get more information about how the decision was made. Sound as if she cares for the patient.

5. Uncertainty and conflict A B C (D) E

What was good?
Offer to talk to clinicians. Valid point about media not dictating decisions made by health organisation.
What could be improved?
Dismissive/unhelpful. No mention of resources issue. Offer to work together/look at options to deal with situations. Defensive manner. No attempt made to talk to chair. Sound less defensive. Give more potential avenues for information/intelligence gathering. Need to sound like you care about the patient. Defended the norm – not responding to exceptional claim.

Scenario 6: Breast screening uptake rates

General performance

What was good?
Generally the candidate seemed to understand the material and demonstrated experience working in this area.
What could be improved? Very nervous throughout. Poor start with no introduction. Lots of 'ums', pauses and uncertainties before each reply. Needs to make eye contact and sound confident.
Key tip for candidate: it is important to go into the exam confident. You only have 8 minutes so you do not have the luxury of easing yourself into the situation. Build up confidence by doing a number of mocks so the process becomes second nature, volunteer for visible roles during service work (e.g. chairing meetings, media work) and before each scenario prepare your short introduction/welcome so you can have a strong beginning to build off.

1. **Presenting communication** A B C (D) E

What was good?
Clear on table and 'we have a graph'. Avoided jargon.
What could be improved? Mumbled. Appeared very nervous (especially at the beginning). Poorly presented. Hesitant. Not much eye contact. Need to be more confident. Needs better body language. Avoid sounding like you don't know what you are talking about. No introduction/clarity of meeting. Stop fiddling with paper.

2. **Listening and comprehending** A B (C) D E

What was good?
Did look at examiner and maintained good eye contact. Answered all questions posed.
What could be improved? Responded with uncertainty: 'Oh I don't know'. Sighing, paper fiddling, constant use of information on paper. Limited/little info provided. Ignored audience. Take clues from body language, tone, etc.

3. Assimilating relevant information A B C (D) E

What was good?
Variation in rates discussed, even if briefly.
What could be improved?
Could give some information on screening. Did not explain role of GPs (minimal) or how they might be supported to increase uptake – or other community measures to improve screening uptake. No answer given as to why rates declining. Extremely limited discussion of just about everything. Talked about practices but initially no ideas as to why uptake varied. '70% OK because government says so' – better explanation as to why rates might vary needed.

4. Reasoning, analytical and judgement A B C (D) E

What was good?
Appeared to understand wider context. Mentioned 'set against other priorities' versus benefits/costs. Raised issue that if uptake increased would need to ensure rest of system could cope.
What could be improved?
Build on benefits articulated. No concept of looking at practices as a whole. Planned to share practice data between practices. Not clear as to why some practices poorly performing and others better performing. Be clear as to what data can be shared with whom. Think more widely about what might be reasons why rates are low from both practice and population perspective.

5. Uncertainty and conflict A B (C) D E

What was good?
Content good. Summarised well. Offered to undertake further work. Would aim to make intervention cost neutral and look at issue practice by practice.
What could be improved?
Positive message but delivered in a very negative way. Mentioned financial incentives but not in any coherent detail. Provide more information. Explain answers properly.

Scenario 7: Emergency hospital admissions

General performance

What was good? Lots of advice, good points and ideas to use the data.
What could be improved? Clearer message – initially unconvincing that they understood the data and be clear over concepts of significance.
Key tip for candidate: most scenarios have data in them and a key skill is quickly understanding and summarising this information to someone else. Practise summarising tables and graphs to a friend or family member who has no background in public health.

1. **Presenting communication** (A) B C D E

What was good? Confident introduction. Lots of positive and no significant negative. Clear and confident presentation of facts. No jargon. Appropriate to audience. Good engagement. Maintained good eye contact.
What could be improved? Style was perhaps a bit 'ploddy' when going through the data but really a minor point.

2. **Listening and comprehending** (A) B C D E

What was good? Lots of positive and no significant negative. Answered all questions comprehensively and in an appropriate manner. Active listening.
What could be improved? Some of the responses in the first half of the scenario could perhaps have been expanded on and so been clearer.

3. Assimilating relevant information A B C (D) E

What was good?
Went systematically through the data and improved a little as the scenario played out.
What could be improved?
Got significance all wrong and muddled. Thought that data from residential and care homes showed no difference. Discussion limited of presenting data and changes over time. Although covered most of the detail of the data, did not inspire confidence regarding the interpretation of the data, e.g. confused about confidence intervals and limited interpretation. Could have covered issues such as the difference between rates and absolute numbers.

4. Reasoning, analytical and judgement A B (C) D E

What was good?
Proxy factors mentioned. Need for age standardisation mentioned. Percentage change covered. Need for improved data, trend analysis, etc. to get more comparable results. Commented on the fact that other quality issues were potentially important.
What could be improved?
Could have covered year-on-year changes. Limited discussion as to how useful the data provided is in explaining the local context and the role of the task force. Potential issue regarding small sample size not mentioned. Increased discussion as to what to do with non-home people since the task group does not cover them. Not clear on treatment issues. Could have discussed strength or otherwise of the evidence and highlighted the difficulty of predicting future performance. Could have discussed the relative performance of the region compared to nationally.

5. Uncertainty and conflict A B (C) D E

What was good?
Mentioned other anecdotal proxy quality factors such as prescribing and more nursing homes – might alter rates.
What could be improved?
Limited discussion as to what the role of the task group was in relation to the figures. More discussion as to how role of the group could be analysed by looking formally at other factors rather than relying on anecdotes. Should avoid too readily accepting potential explanations hypothesised by the role player.

Scenario 8: Smoking ban

General performance

What was good? Tried to make the most of providing public health information to inform the article that was going to be written.
What could be improved? A stronger defence of the evidence and ensuring that any of the reporter's misconceptions were addressed before the end of the scenario.
Key tip for candidate: while trying to be helpful and show empathy, candidates can often be reluctant to contradict the role player and avoid conflict. However, it is important to stand your ground and not to fall into the trap of leading questions. Be polite and show understanding of the role player's position, but if you do not agree with a particular viewpoint it is better to state this and be clear about your opinion.

1. **Presenting communication** A B (C) D E

What was good? Reasonable start/introduction. Introduced himself. Had sent information. Used appropriate language. Checked journalist had data. Did some reasonable signposting. Reasonably calm and clear. Tried to make the most of providing public health information to inform the article that was going to be written.
What could be improved? Too much detail – started talking early on about confidence intervals and p values, which only confused the issue instead of made easier to understand aspects. Clarity about purpose/message of interview. Long pauses after questions posed. Seemed to forget he was talking to a journalist at times. Used statistical terms without always explaining them. Be clear who the audience is and reply appropriately.

2. **Listening and comprehending** A (B) C D E

What was good? Appropriate manner. Answered questions posed in appropriate manner and in totality.
What could be improved? Appeared to want to please journalist rather than clarity about own position. Appeasement appeared sympathetic to opponents of ban. Clarity on message/purpose. What message did the candidate wish to be reported? More active listening to lead to fewer pauses.

3. Assimilating relevant information A B C (D) E

What was good?
Covered results and described much of the data well but seemed unimpressed with reduction. Discussed multi-faceted approach to smoking reduction. Importance of protecting workers covered.
What could be improved?
State facts without giving opinions when talking to journalists. Poor understanding of ban/use of data evidence/context. Failed to discuss aspects of data on salivary cotinine levels which supported ban. Did not identify possible selection bias in the questionnaire data.

4. Reasoning, analytical and judgement A B C (D) E

What was good?
Mentioned lung cancer/increase in food sales in pubs due to ban. Covered issue regarding secondary smoke. Tried to pacify reporter about smoking areas in pubs, though limited success.
What could be improved?
Should have better dealt with methodological limitations of the three studies. Little judgement/rationale/context. 'I will send over details for smoking cessation services' – should have had contact details to hand/clear rationale. Did not fully explore issues (good and bad) with the data/study design. More detail on study design and how it could be improved if done again.

5. Uncertainty and conflict A B C (D) E

What was good?
Asked to see draft of report. Supportive of local research and did not just discuss concerns raised about negative aspects of the ban. Responded to issues with business with some empathy, though limited success. Reasonable signposting. Did not identify that business performance could be improved due to a more pleasant environment.
What could be improved?
Stronger defence based on evidence. Readily conceded to journalist's points about data and sympathy for smokers having to be outside. Caved in. Not holding the public health line. Undermined confidence in study by stating he expected reduction to be higher. Accentuate the positive when technical evidence is limited. Did not emphasise weaknesses and strengths of the research.

Glossary

Term	Definition	Lay communication/context-specific example
Absolute risk reduction	The difference in the rate of adverse events in exposed and unexposed groups. This is mathematically identical to the *attributable risk* for a risk factor. (cf *relative risk reduction* and *preventable fraction*)	Suppose the risk of a deep vein thrombosis reduces from 0.03% to 0.02% following stopping the oral contraceptive pill; the absolute risk reduction is 0.01%, or 1 in 10,000.
Accuracy	The closeness of a measured value to a standard or known value. (cf *precision*)	The measurements of blood pressure in a patient by 10 different students were very precise as there was little variation in the results. However, all the readings were about 10 mmHg greater than the true blood pressure due to an inaccurate sphygmomanometer.
Attack rate	The proportion of those individuals who are at risk of an infectious disease who become clinically ill in a given time period (usually expressed as a percentage).	In an outbreak of food poisoning, out of 1000 diners there were 50 cases of diarrhoea within a week of the meal. The attack rate was 50 out of 1000 diners, or 5% of diners were affected.
Attributable fraction	The proportion of an outcome in people exposed that is due entirely to the risk factor (the *attributable risk* divided by the risk in the exposed population). (cf *preventable fraction* and *relative risk reduction*)	If smokers have a 25.2% lifetime risk of lung cancer and non-smokers a 0.2% lifetime risk, the attributable fraction is (25.2% – 0.2% = 25% divided by the risk in the exposed population (25.2%) = 0.99 (99%), or 99 out of 100 lung cancers in smokers are due to smoking.
Attributable risk	The difference in the rate of disease in the exposed group as compared to the unexposed group. This is mathematically identical to the *absolute risk reduction* for the effect of a treatment.	If smokers have a 25.2% lifetime risk of lung cancer and non-smokers a 0.2% lifetime risk, the risk of lung cancer in smokers that is attributable to, or caused by, their smoking is 25.2% – 0.2% = 25%.

(Continued)

Term	Definition	Lay communication/context-specific example
Basic reproduction number (R_0)	The average number of individuals directly infected by an infectious case during the entire infectious period when entering a totally susceptible population. (cf *effective reproductive number* and *secondary attack rate*)	If the basic reproduction number (R_0) of measles is 12, each case of measles introduced into a non-immune population would result in the infection of 12 other people.
Clinically significant	An effect that is large enough that it is worth treating a patient. (cf *statistically significant*)	A new blood pressure drug reduces diastolic blood pressure by 0.001 mmHg. Although the result from the trial was statistically significant, the effect is not clinically significant because it is so small and does not warrant widespread use of the drug (which may have negative clinical consequences like side effects).
Confidence interval (CI)	A calculated interval with a given probability (usually 95%) that the true value of the effect lies within the interval.	Suppose the increased risk of lung cancer from radon exposure is 20% and the 95% confidence interval is 16%–24%. Therefore we can be 95% confident that the true increased risk lies between 16% and 24%, and conversely, there is a 5% (or 1 in 20) chance that the true risk lies outside this range.
Confounding variable	A factor that is independently associated with the exposure and outcome/disease under study, but is not an intermediate factor between exposure and outcome.	People who eat more fruits and vegetables are less likely to be obese. However, this observation may be confounded (or explained either completely or partly) by people who eat more fruits and vegetables also being more likely to take exercise, which is independently related to obesity.
Cost-benefit analysis	A formal comparison of the costs and outcomes of alternative interventions of which the costs and effects are not equal and results are expressed in terms of net benefit. Both costs and outcomes are measured in monetary units.	The cost-benefit analysis estimates that through savings over the next 20 years, investing £5 million in new road surfaces would benefit the economy by £10 million, compared to a £15 million benefit from investing £5 million in recruiting more nurses.
Cost-effectiveness analysis	A formal comparison of the costs and outcomes of alternative interventions of which the costs and consequences are not equal and the results are expressed in terms of cost per unit of outcome. Outcomes are measured in natural units.	When comparing two blood pressure-lowering drugs, the cost-effectiveness analysis shows that drug A costs £5 per mmHg reduction in systolic blood pressure, compared to £4 per mmHg reduction for drug B.

(*Continued*)

Term	Definition	Lay communication/context-specific example
Cost-minimisation analysis	Compares the costs of alternative interventions that are assumed to have an equivalent effect. The goal is to find the least costly alternative.	Using a cost-minimisation analysis, nurse-led endoscopy units may have been shown to cost £60 more per patient than doctor-led units.
Cost-utility analysis	A formal comparison of the costs and outcomes of alternative interventions of which the costs and consequences are not equal and the results are expressed in terms of cost per unit of outcome. Outcomes are usually measured in *quality-adjusted life years* (QALYs).	Per patient, the benefit (in terms of gain in quality-adjusted life years) from repairing a ruptured abdominal aortic aneurysm is significantly greater than prescribing a walking stick for recurrent falls (that also has a health benefit). However, the cost per QALY is much greater for the abdominal aortic aneurysm repair, as for the price of one operation you could buy more than 1000 walking sticks.
Cumulative incidence	See *risk*.	
Effective (net) reproductive number	The average number of individuals directly infected by an infectious case during the entire infectious period when entering a typical population of susceptible and non-susceptible individuals. (cf *basic reproduction number* and *secondary attack rate*)	Each case of measles ($R_0 = 12$) introduced into a population half of whom were immune to measures would result in the infection of six other people.
Endemic	The maintenance of a disease or illness in a community or region without the need for external inputs.	Herpes simplex virus is endemic to the UK; it does not require any external increase in cases to be maintained. This compares to malaria, which can be acquired in the UK in some exceptional scenarios but is not maintained due to lack of vector.
Epidemic	The occurrence in a community or region of cases of a disease or illness clearly in excess of normal expectancy.	A 'flu epidemic is declared when the number of cases identified is greater than what would be expected under usual circumstances.
Evidence-based medicine	The ability to access, summarise and apply information from the literature to day-to-day clinical problems.	Evidence-based medicine is decision making based on sound scientific study rather than on the opinion of one or more individuals.
False negative	Test result is negative but the person has the disease (i.e. test result is incorrect).	A test result that indicates no disease but in fact the person does have the disease.
False positive	Test result is positive but the person does not have the disease (i.e. test result is incorrect).	A test result that indicates disease but in fact the person does not have the disease.

(Continued)

Term	Definition	Lay communication/context-specific example
Gross domestic product (GDP)	GDP measures total output within the geographical boundaries of the country, regardless of the nationality of the entities producing the output.	In 2012, the GDP of the United States was \$16,250 billion and for Monaco \$6 billion. The GDP per capita, however, was \$160,000 for Monaco and \$50,000 for the United States.
Hazard	A source of potential damage, harm or adverse health effects (cf *risk*).	The danger associated with something.
Herd immunity threshold	The proportion of the population who need to be immune to put transmission in decline.	Once 95% of children are vaccinated against measles, the disease no longer has a large enough susceptible population in which to sustain replication and case numbers will then decline.
Incremental cost-effectiveness ratio (ICER)	The ICER is obtained by dividing the cost differences (C1 – C2) by the outcome differences (E1 – E2) for an intervention where C1 and E1 are cost and effect of the intervention, and C2 and E2 are cost and effect of the control (or current practice).	Suppose a person with pancreatic cancer is expected to live for 12 months following diagnosis with a quality of life score of 0.4 (0.4 × 12 months = 0.4 QALYs) and a drug that costs £36,000 can increase life expectancy by 12 months with a quality of life score of 0.8 (0.8 × 24 months = 1.6 QALYs). C1 – C2 = £50,000 and E1 – E2 = 1.6 QALYs – 0.4 QALYs. Therefore ICER = £36,000/1.2 QALYs = £30,000/QALY.
Incidence	The number of new cases or events during a specified time period.	In 2011, the incidence of lung cancer among males in the UK was 77 new cases per 100,000 males.
Incidence density	See *rate*.	
Incidence rate	See *rate*.	
Incidence risk	See *risk*.	
Incubation period	The time interval between acquisition of an infectious agent and the appearance of the first sign or symptom of the disease.	The incubation period for measles is around 7–12 days; following exposure, it will take 7–12 days before any symptoms appear.
Infectious period	The time interval during which transmission to a susceptible host is possible.	Measles is infectious from about 4 days before the rash appears to about 4 days after it goes; this is the infectious period.
Latent period	The time interval between acquisition of an infectious agent and the onset of infectiousness.	For measles it can take 7–12 days before a rash appears following an infection and measles is infectious from about 4 days before the rash appears so the latent period for measles is around 3–8 days.

(Continued)

Term	Definition	Lay communication/context-specific example
Likelihood ratio (LR) of test results	Likelihood ratio of a negative test (LR–): A ratio of odds of disease given a negative test result to the pre-test odds of disease. Likelihood ratio of a positive test (LR+): A ratio of the odds of disease given a positive test result to the pre-test odds of disease.	The LR describes how the odds of a patient having a disease change based on the results of a test. A LR of 1 suggests the test adds no information. A LR– much lower than 1 suggests that a negative test is helpful in excluding the disease. A LR+ much higher than 1 suggests that a positive test result is helpful in confirming the disease Post-test odds = pre-test odds × likelihood ratio
Mortality	Death.	
Morbidity	Disease.	
Negative predictive value (NPV)	The proportion of patients with a negative test result who do not have the disease. (cf *positive predictive value*)	Suppose following a prostate-specific antigen (PSA) test with a cut-off at 4.0 ng/mL, 85% of men tested with a negative test don't have the disease, and 15% (about 1 in 7 men with a negative result) do despite the negative result. The NPV is 85%.
Number needed to treat (NNT)	The number of patients who must be treated in order to prevent one adverse event. This is the reciprocal of the *absolute risk reduction*.	If to prevent one heart attack, 60 people with no known heart disease have to be treated with statins for 5 years, the NNT to prevent one heart attack would be 60.
Odds	The odds of disease is the number of people with disease divided by the number without disease.	If out of every 10 people exposed to severe carbon monoxide poisoning, one person dies, the odds of death from severe carbon monoxide poisoning is 1/9, or 0.11. By comparison, the risk is 1/10, or 0.10.
Odds ratio (OR)	The ratio of the odds of exposure in cases compared to the odds of exposure in controls (exposure OR). Or The ratio of the odds of disease in the exposed group compared to the odds of disease in the unexposed (disease OR). *Note*: Odds ratios will approximate the risk ratio when the disease is rare. Where the disease is common, the odds ratio will always be more extreme than the risk ratio, so the value of the odds ratio should not be used to communicate relative risk. (cf *risk ratio*)	Odds of exposure in the cases divided by the odds of exposure in the controls. If OR: >1: An increased risk of the outcome in exposed. =1: No difference in risk of the outcome in exposed compared to unexposed. <1: A decreased risk of the outcome in exposed.

(*Continued*)

Term	Definition	Lay communication/context-specific example
Opportunity cost	Within the context of a rationed system, this is what can no longer be funded when a decision is made to fund something else.	The opportunity of cost of funding a new weight management service is that a dietary education campaign has to be scrapped.
p value	The probability that an effect as least as extreme as that observed in a study could have occurred by chance alone. By convention, a *p* value less than 0.05 is taken to mean that the effect is *statistically significant*.	A trial shows that a new blood pressure drug reduces diastolic blood pressure by 5 mmHg with a *p* value of 0.03. There is therefore a 3% (0.03 as a percentage) chance that the reduction may have occurred by chance and a 97% chance that the drug truly reduces diastolic blood pressure. This is less than 0.05 and therefore defined as statistically significant.
Pandemic	An epidemic occurring worldwide or over a very wide area, crossing international boundaries, and usually affecting a large number of people.	A viral haemorrhagic fever pandemic is declared when more cases occur than expected in different countries and parts of the world.
Population attributable fraction (PAF)	Measure of the benefit of eliminating exposure from entire population as a percentage reduction in the outcome, calculated by dividing the *population attributable risk* by the incidence in the population.	If smokers have a 25.2% lifetime risk of lung cancer and non-smokers a 0.2% lifetime risk, and 20% of the population smoke, then 25.2%*20% + 0.2%*80% = 5.2% of the population will develop lung cancer; then the population attributable fraction is the population attributable risk (see below, 5%)/5.2% = 99%, or 99% of lung cancer cases would not happen if no one smoked.
Population attributable risk (PAR)	Measure of the benefit of eliminating exposure from entire population. Calculated either by multiplying *attributable risk* by the proportion of exposed individuals in the population or by subtracting the disease incidence in the unexposed population from the total disease incidence in the population.	If 20% of the population smoke and the attributable risk of lung cancer from smoking is 25% over a lifetime, then the population attributable risk of lung cancer due to smoking is the attributable risk (25%)*20% = 5%, or 5 out of 100 people in the population would not get lung cancer if no one smoked.
Positive predictive value (PPV)	The proportion of patients with a positive test result who truly have the disease. (cf *negative predictive value*)	Suppose following a PSA test with a cut-off at 4.0 ng/mL, 30% of men tested with a positive test have the disease, and 70% (about 7 in 10 men with a positive result) do not despite the positive result. The PPV is 30%.

(Continued)

Term	Definition	Lay communication/context-specific example
Post-test probability	The probability that a patient has a disease after a diagnostic test has been carried out. This is identical to the positive predictive value (if the test result was +ve). (cf *pre-test probability*)	Suppose around 20% of men aged over 65 have prostate cancer – the pre-test probability of having prostate cancer is 20%, or 1 in 5. Following a PSA test with a cut-off at 4.0 ng/mL, 30% of men tested with a positive test have the disease, and 70% (about 7 in 10 men with a positive result) do not despite the positive result. The post-test probability of having prostate cancer with a positive test is 30%.
Purchasing power parity (PPP)	To compare living standards across countries, PPP exchange rates are constructed by comparing the national prices for a large basket of goods and services. These rates are used to translate different currencies into a common currency to measure the purchasing power of per capita income in different countries.	1 U.S. dollar (USD) will buy you a lot more in India than in America. Using the USD as a common currency unit, in 2012 the GDP measured as PPP per capita in India is 5140 USD compared to a gross GDP per capita of 1490 USD. These both compare to a GDP per capita (both PPP and gross) in the United States of about 50,000 USD.
Precision	The closeness of two or more measurements to each other (independent of accuracy). (cf *accuracy*)	The measurements of blood pressure in a patient by 10 different students were very precise, as there was little variation in the results. However, all the readings were about 10 mmHg greater than the true blood pressure due to an inaccurate sphygmomanometer.
Pre-test probability	The probability that a patient has a disease before the diagnostic test has been carried out. This is the equivalent of the prevalence of the disease in people with the same clinical features as the index patient. (cf *post-test probability*)	Suppose around 20% of men aged over 65 have prostate cancer – the pre-test probability of having prostate cancer is 20%, or 1 in 5. Following a PSA test with a cut-off at 4.0 ng/mL, 30% of men tested with a positive test have the disease, and 70% (about 7 in 10 men with a positive result) do not despite the positive result. The post-test probability of having prostate cancer with a positive test is 30%.
Prevalence	The proportion of individuals in a population with a disease or condition at a given time.	The prevalence of lung cancer among UK adult males was about 85 per 100,000 in 2006.

(*Continued*)

Term	Definition	Lay communication/context-specific example
Preventable fraction	The proportion of the population who would be prevented from an outcome if exposed to an intervention compared to if not exposed (used when the exposure is protective). This is mathematically identical to the *relative risk reduction*.	Assume 10% of bicycle accidents involving cyclists who are not wearing a helmet result in serious head injury, and that wearing bicycle helmets reduces this risk to 4%. The preventable fraction = absolute risk reduction/event rate. This is (10% – 4%)/10% = 60%; among those cycling without helmets, 60% of serious head injuries resulting from bicycle accidents are preventable by the cyclist wearing a helmet. This is the same as 1 – RR (relative risk).
Quality-adjusted life year (QALY)	QALYs incorporate both the quantity and quality of life dimensions. They are calculated by estimating the total life years gained from a treatment and weighting each year with a quality of life score (from 0, representing worst health, to 1, representing best health) to reflect the quality of life in that year.	Suppose a person with pancreatic cancer is expected to live for 12 months following diagnosis with a quality of life score of 0.4 and a drug can increase life expectancy by 12 months with a quality of life score of 0.8. The increase in QALYs gained by taking the drug is: (2 years × 0.8) – (1 year × 0.4) = 1.6 QALYs – 0.4 QALYs = 1.2 QALYs
Rate	The frequency at which an event occurs in a defined time period in a given population. Often expressed as number of events per total person-time at risk of developing disease. (Also called the *incidence rate*, *incidence density*, or force of morbidity/mortality.)	In 2006, the rate of lung cancer in newer smokers aged 40–79 was about 15 cases per 100,000 person years.
Rate ratio	The ratio of the rate of disease in exposed group compared to the rate of disease in the unexposed group.	>1: An increased disease rate in exposed compared to the unexposed. =1: No difference in disease rate in exposed compared to unexposed. <1: A decreased disease rate in exposed compared to unexposed. *Note*: A rate ratio can be quantified when communicated; i.e. RR of 2 is double the disease rate, RR of 0.5 is half, or a 50% reduction.
Relative risk (RR)	A collective term for the ratio measures of association, including *risk ratio*, *rate ratio*, *hazard ratio* and *odds ratio*.	Probability of having an outcome among the exposed compared to the unexposed (i.e. divide the two risks). >1: An increased risk of an outcome in exposed compared to the unexposed.

(*Continued*)

Term	Definition	Lay communication/context-specific example
		=1: No difference in risk of an outcome in exposed compared to unexposed. <1: A decreased risk of an outcome in exposed compared to unexposed.
Relative risk reduction (RRR)	The reduction in adverse events achieved by removing an exposure, expressed as a proportion of the baseline rate. (cf *preventable fraction* and *attributable fraction*)	The absolute risk reduction (ARR) as a percentage of the total risk in the population. Suppose the risk of a deep vein thrombosis reduces from 0.02% to 0.01% when stopping the oral contraceptive pill; the ARR is 0.02 – 0.01% = 0.01%, and the relative risk reduction = ARR/event rate = 0.01%/0.02% = 50%, or half the risk. This can also be calculated as 1 – RR (relative risk).
Reliability	Describes how well a test will produce the same result when repeated a number of times. (cf *validity*)	A reliable test will produce similar results on repeated testing of the same outcome.
Repeatability	The variation in repeat measurements made on the same subject under identical conditions.	The repeatability of a test is a way of assessing its reliability.
Risk	The probability that an event will occur within a stated period of time (also called *cumulative incidence* or *incidence risk*).	The lifetime risk of lung cancer is about 6%, or 6 out of 100 people will get lung cancer at some point in their lives.
Risk ratio	The ratio of the risk of disease in the exposed group compared to risk of disease in the unexposed group.	>1: An increased risk of an outcome in exposed compared to the unexposed. =1: No difference in risk of an outcome in exposed compared to unexposed. <1: A decreased risk of an outcome in exposed compared to unexposed. *Note*: For a risk ratio, the risk can be quantified; i.e. RR of 2 is double the risk, RR of 0.5 is half the risk, or a 50% reduction.
Secondary attack rate	The proportion of individuals in contact with infectious cases who become (clinically) ill (usually expressed as a percentage). (cf *basic reproductive number* and *effective reproductive number*)	When a resident infected with a new strain of 'flu virus entered a care home, 10 out of 100 current residents became unwell with 'flu. The secondary attack rate was 10/100, or 10%.

(*Continued*)

Term	Definition	Lay communication/context-specific example
Sensitivity	The proportion of patients with a disease who have a positive test result. (cf *specificity*)	Suppose the sensitivity of a PSA test with a cut-off at 4.0 ng/mL is 21%; therefore 21% of men tested who have prostate cancer have a positive test result, and 79% of men tested who have prostate cancer have a false negative result. Unlike positive and negative predictive values, the sensitivity and specificity of a test do not change with population disease prevalence.
Specificity	The proportion of patients without a disease who have a negative test result. (cf *sensitivity*)	Suppose the specificity of a PSA test with a cut-off at 4.0 ng/mL is 91%; therefore 91% of men tested who do not have prostate cancer have a negative test result, and 9% of men tested who do not have prostate cancer have a false positive result. Unlike positive and negative predictive values, the sensitivity and specificity of a test do not change with population disease prevalence.
Statistically significant	An effect that is unlikely to have occurred by chance; by convention, this is commonly defined as having an associated *p* value of less than 0.05. (cf *clinically significant*)	A trial shows that a new blood pressure drug reduces diastolic blood pressure by 5 mmHg with a *p* value of 0.03. There is therefore a 3% (0.03 as a percentage) chance that the reduction may have occurred by chance and a 97% chance that the drug truly reduces diastolic blood pressure. This is less than 0.05 and therefore defined as statistically significant.
Statistical neighbours	Comparator organisations that are deemed suitable for benchmarking against your local population because of demographic similarities, such as age, socio-economic structure or numbers of students.	Comparing the health of our population to a statistical neighbour helps us identify whether the health of our population is better or worse than we would expect given our population make-up.
Vaccine efficacy	Vaccine efficacy is the difference in disease *attack rate* between vaccinated and unvaccinated populations, divided by the *attack rate* in the unvaccinated population, expressed as a percentage.	Vaccine efficacy is the percentage reduction in people who become unwell in a group of vaccinated people compared to those who are unvaccinated. If 10% of people without a flu vaccine become unwell compared to 1% of those with a vaccine, the vaccine is ((10% – 1%)/10%) = 90% efficacious.
Validity	Describes how much a tool measures what it intends to measure. (cf *reliability*)	A valid questionnaire for depression distinguishes the presence or absence of depression, rather than other affective disorders.

References

Acheson D. 1988. Public Health in England. The report of the Committee of Inquiry into the future development to the Public Health Function. London: HMSO Command Paper 289.

Adair J. 1973. *Action-Centred Leadership*. New York: McGraw-Hill.

Beattie A. 1991. Knowledge and control in health promotion: A test case for social policy and social theory. In Gabe J, Calnan M, Bury M (eds.), *The Sociology of the Health Service*. London: Routledge. pp. 162–202.

Bennis W, Nanus B. 1985. Leaders: *The Strategies for Taking Charge*. New York: Harper & Row.

Bradshaw JR. 1972. The taxonomy of social need. In MacLachlan G (ed.), *Problems and Progress in Medical Care*. Oxford: Oxford University Press. pp. 69–82.

Dahlgren G, Whitehead M. 1991. *Policies and Strategies to Promote Social Equity in Health*. Stockholm, Sweden: Institute for Futures Studies. http://www.iffs.se/wp-content/uploads/2011/01/20080109110739filmZ8UVQv2wQFShMRF6cuT.pdf.

Davison I, Cooper R, Bullock A. 2010. The objective structured public health examination: A study of reliability using multi-level analysis. *Medical Teacher* 32, 582–585.

Department for Education and Skills. 2006. *Teenage Pregnancy: Accelerating the Strategy to 2010*. London: DfES.

Ghate D, Lewis J, Welbourn, D. 2013. Systems leadership: Exceptional leadership for exceptional times – Synthesis paper. Available from www.virtualstaffcollege.co.uk

Goleman D. 1995. *Emotional Intelligence – Why It Can Matter More Than IQ*. London: Bloomsbury Publishing.

Greenhalgh T. 2014. *How to Read a Paper: The Basics of Evidence Based Medicine*. 5th ed. London: Wiley-Blackwell.

Griffiths S, Jewell T, Donnelly P. 2005. Public health in practice: The three domains of public health. *Public Health* 119, 907–913.

Heller R. 1998. *DK Essential Managers: Managing Change*. New York: DK Adult.

Hersey P, Blanchard K. 1977. *Management of Organizational Behavior – Utilizing Human Resources*. 3rd ed. Englewood Cliffs, NJ: Prentice Hall.

Herzberg F. 1968. One More Time: How Do You Motivate Employees? *Harvard Business Review*. 46(1), 53–62.

Hochbaum GM. 1958. *Public Participation in Medical Screening Programs: A Socio-Psychological Study*. PHS no. 572. Washington, DC: U.S. Government Printing Office.

Kotter J. 1995. *Leading Change*. Boston: Harvard Business Review Press.

Kotter J. 2011. Change Management vs. Change Leadership – What's the Difference? *Forbes* [online].

Kubler-Ross E. 1969. *On Death and Dying*. New York: Macmillan.

Lewin K. 1947. Frontiers of group dynamics: Concept, method and reality in social science, social equilibria, and social change. *Human Relations* 1, 5–41.

Lewis G, Sheringham J, Lopez Bernal J, Crayford T. 2014. *Mastering Public Health: A Postgraduate Guide to Examinations and Revalidation*, 2nd ed. Boca Raton, FL: CRC Press.

McGregor D. 1960. *The Human Side of Enterprise*. New York: McGraw Hill.

Mintzberg H. 1975. The manager's job: Folklore and fact. *Harvard Business Review* 53(4), 49–61.

National Audit Office. 2014. *NAO Model of Commissioning and the Third Sector*. London: National Audit Office.

NHS Improving Quality. 2013. NHS change model. http://www.nhsiq.nhs.uk/capacity-capability/nhs-change-model.aspx.

Nuffield Council on Bioethics. 2007. *Public Health: Ethical Issues*. London: Nuffield Council on Bioethics. http://nuffieldbioethics.org/wp-content/uploads/2014/07/Public-health-ethicalissues.pdf.

Oswald M, Cox D, on behalf of the RCGP Ethics Committee. 2011. *Making Difficult Choices: Ethical Commissioning Guidance to General Practitioners*. London: Royal College of General Practitioners.

Prochaska JO, DiClemente CC. 1984. Self-change processes, self-efficacy and decisional balance across five stages of smoking cessation. In *Advances in Cancer Control – 1983*. Engstrom PF, Anderson PN, Mortenson LE (eds.). New York: Alan R. Liss. pp. 131–140.

Public Health Ontario. 2013. The eight steps to developing healthy public policy. Ontario: Public Health Ontario.

Roberts A, Marshall L, Charlesworth A. 2012. *A Decade of Austerity*. London: Nuffield Trust.

Rogow F et al. 2008. *Unnatural Causes*. Discussion Guide. San Francisco: California Newsreel.

Salovey P, Mayer JD. 1990. Emotional intelligence. *Imagination, Cognition, and Personality* 9, 185–211.

Steiner C. 1997. *Achieving Emotional Literacy*. New York: Avon.

Stevens A, Gabby J. 1991. Needs assessment needs assessment. *Health Trends* 23(1), 20–23.

Taylor F. 1911. *The Principles of Scientific Management*. New York: Harper.

Thaler RH, Sunstein CR. 2008. *Nudge: Improving Decisions about Health, Wealth and Happiness*. New Haven, CT: Yale University Press.

Turner A. 2012. Tips for being first amongst equals – Leadership from within a partnership. *Health Service Journal*, July, 30–32.

Wanless D. 2004. *Securing Good Health for the Whole Population: Final Report – February 2004*. London: Department of Health.

World Health Organisation. 1986. The Ottawa charter for health promotion. First International Conference on Health Promotion, Ottawa, November 21, 1986. WHO/HPR/HEP/95.1. Geneva: WHO.

World Health Organisation. 2014. The HIA procedure. Geneva: WHO. http://www.who.int/hia/tools/process/en/.

Index

Note: Locator with italic *f* denotes Figure. Locator with italic *t* denotes Table.

A

Absolute risk reduction (ARR), 175, 183
Accuracy, 3, 175
Action learning sets (ALSs), 73
Attack rate, 175
Attributable fraction, 175
Attributable risk, 175

B

Basic reproduction number (R0), 176
Beattie typology model, 23–24, 25*f*
Bioethics intervention ladder, 24*f*
Brief interventions, 24

C

Cancer screening, 15
Centre for Evidence Based Medicine (CEBM), 50
Certificate of completion of training (CCT), 88
Change management, 67, 73
  assessment tool, 79–80
  change models, 74
  force field analysis, 75
  gap analysis, 74
  history of, 68
  influencing people, 79–80, 81
  Kotter's eight-step model, 75–77
  Kubler-Ross's stages of change, 78*f*
  meetings, 81–82
  motivation, 77
  motivator and hygiene factors, 78*t*
  NHS change model, 77, 78*f*
  project management, 83
  public health priorities and policies, 82–83
  reaction to change, 77, 79
  stages of change, 74–75
  theory X and theory Y, 68
Change models, 74
  stages of, 30*f*
Chemical, biological, radiological or nuclear (CBRN) events, 13
Chemical meteorology (CHEMET), 14
Clinically significant, 176
Commissioning cycle, 33
Communication
  during decontamination, 14
  during outbreaks, 11
  grid, 6*t*
  in healthcare public health, 59
  non-verbal, 39–40
  OSPHE tips, 90
  risk, 7–8
  skills, 2, 3–7
Community, 29
Confidence interval (CI), 62, 176
Confounding variable, 176
Cost-benefit analysis (CBA), 176
Cost effectiveness analysis (CEA), 176
Cost minimisation analysis (CMA), 177
Cost-utility analysis (CUA), 177
Critical Appraisal Skills Programme (CASP), 50
Cycle for developing healthy public policy, 28*f*

D

Dahlgren and Whitehead's health rainbow, 22*f*
Data interpretation, 51
Diagnostic related groups (DRGs), 51
Directly standardised rates (DSRs), 61
Disease distribution pattern, 12*f*, 13*f*; *see also* Health protection

E

Effective communication, 3
Effective (net) reproductive number, 177
Emergency operation centre (EOC), 13

Emergency prevention preparedness and response (EPPR), 2, 13–14
Emotional awareness, 40
Emotional intelligence, 80
Emotional literacy, 40
Endemic, 177
Epidemic, 177
Evidence-based medicine, 177

F

Faculty of Public Health (FPH) of the Royal Colleges of Physicians, 87
False negative, 177
False positive, 177
Force field analysis, 75

G

Gap analysis, 74; *see also* Change management
General Medical Council (GMC), 91
General practitioner (GP), 34, 89
Grading of Recommendations Assessment, Development and Evaluation (GRADE), 50
Gross domestic product (GDP), 178

H

Hazard, 178
Health belief model, 32*t*, 43
Healthcare Leadership Model, 71
Healthcare public health, 45
- challenges, 46
- communication challenges in, 59–65
- data interpretation, 51–52
- friends and family test outcomes, 64
- funding pressures on services, 47*f*
- health and social care needs, 47–48
- healthcare system structure, 58–59
- influences of need, supply and demand, 48*f*
- interview on vascular surgical hub, 62–63
- practising, 45–46
- practising public health tip, 46, 49, 50, 52
- prioritisation, 48, 49
- programme budgeting, 50
- responding to scarcity, 48–51
- strategic decision making, 52–54
- SWOT analysis, 54, 58
- variation in surgical procedure rates, 61

Healthcare resource groups (HRGs), 51
Healthcare systems, 58–59
Health impact assessment (HIA), 26, 28*f*
Health needs assessment (HNA), 48
Health promotion, 21, 22
- assimilation of information, 34
- Beattie typology model of, 23–24, 25*f*
- bioethics intervention ladder, 24*f*
- brief interventions, 24
- change model stages, 30
- commissioning cycle, 33
- consulting target population, 34–35
- Dahlgren and Whitehead's health rainbow, 22*f*
- decision making, 23–25
- effecting individual behaviour change, 23
- effective listening, 38
- emotional awareness, 40
- emotional literacy, 40
- evaluation and monitoring, 40
- health belief model, 32, 43
- health service re-orientation, 32–33
- healthy public policy, 26–27
- implementation problems, 38
- initiative, 22–23
- intervention, 25
- literature review, 35
- message for stakeholders, 37–38
- mode of intervention model, 43
- non-verbal communication, 39
- nudges, 26
- Ottawa Charter for, 42–43
- public health teams, 26, 29, 33
- practising public health tip, 33, 34, 38, 39–40, 42
- readiness to change behaviour, 31*t*
- scenario, 33
- skill development, 29
- stress management, 39–40
- supportive community, 29
- supportive environment, 27, 29
- teenage pregnancy reduction initiative , 41*t*
- teenage pregnancy risk factors, 36*t*
- triggers for health improvement intervention, 34
- uncertainties and conflicts, 37
- understanding your audience, 36

Health protection, 2
- case cluster map, 13
- communication grid, 6*t*
- communication skills, 2, 3–7
- dealing with media, 16–18
- emergency prevention and response, 13–14
- hot zone, 13
- incident command levels, 14
- issues in, 10*t*
- issues with stakeholders, 5*t*
- jargon, 16
- outbreak investigation stages, 11–12
- outbreaks, 8
- pattern of disease cases, 12*f*, 13*f*
- practising public health tip, 3, 4, 6–7, 8, 9, 11, 13, 16, 18, 19
- risk communication, 7–8
- risk of clusters, 12
- risk of screening, 15
- safe situation, 8

screening, 14
social media, 18–19
source-pathway-receptor model, 11*f*
Texas sharpshooter effect, 12
triage, 14
work challenges, 2
zones at an incident, 14*f*
Healthy public policy, 26–27; *see also* Health promotion
cycle for developing, 28*f*
Herd immunity threshold, 178
Hot zone, 13; *see also* Health protection

I

Idea, Development, Exploration, Assessment, Long-Term Follow-Up (IDEAL), 50
Implantable cardiac defibrillators (ICDs), 61
Incident command levels, 14*t*
Incremental costeffectiveness ratio (ICER), 178
Incubation period, 178
Infectious period, 178
Influencing people, 79
Intervention model, 43; *see also* Health promotion

J

Joint strategic needs assessments (JSNAs), 84

K

Kotter's eight-step model, 75–77
Kubler-Ross's stages of change, 78*f*

L

Latent period, 178
Leadership, 67; *see also* Change management; Partnership working
authoritarian, 69
delegative, 69
feedback, 71–72
functional, 69
Healthcare Leadership Model, 71
history of, 68
leadership development, 72–73
managers vs. leaders, 69
mentoring vs. coaching, 73
Myers Briggs type indicator, 71, 72
participative, 70
public health leadership context, 71
practising public health tip, 71, 82, 83
servant, 70
situational, 70
styles, 68
systems, 70
theory X and theory Y, 68
trait theory, 68–69
transactional, 69
transformational, 69
Lifestyle change, 29; *see also* Health promotion
Likelihood ratio (LR), 179
Listening, 38–40

M

Making Every Contact Count (MECC), 24
Managers and leaders, 69
Media, 4, 5*t*, 16–17, 41*t*, 50, 60*t*, 62–63, 81, 82*t*, 89
dealing with, 16–18
social, 18–19
Meeting, preparing, 81
Mode of intervention model, 43
Morbidity, 179
Mortality, 179
Motivation, 77
Multi-source feedback (MSF), 71–72
Myers-Briggs Type Indicator (MBTI), 71, 72

N

National Health Service (NHS), 1, 47, 89; *see also* Change management
change model, 77, 78*f*
National Institute for Health and Care Excellence (NICE), 23, 42, 83
Need, 47
Negative predictive value (NPV), 179
Net reproductive number, 177
Non-verbal communication, 39; *see also* Health promotion
Nudge, 26
Nuffield Council on Bioethics intervention ladder, 24*f*
Number needed to treat (NNT), 179

O

Objective Structured Public Health Examination (OSPHE), 87; *see also* Faculty of Public Health of the Royal Colleges of Physicians
competencies and areas assessed, 88
exam structure and preparation, 89
scenario types, 89
tips, 90–91
video scenarios, 96–97*t*
Odds, 179
Odds ratio (OR), 179
Opportunity cost, 180
Ottawa Charter for Health Promotion, 42–43; *see also* Health promotion
Outbreaks and incidents, 8

P

Packaging the message, 37
Pandemic, 180

Part A Membership of the Faculty of Public Health of the Royal Colleges of Physicians, 87
Part B Membership of the Faculty of Public Health of the Royal Colleges of Physicians, *see* Objective Structured Public Health Examination
Partnership working, 83; *see also* Change management; Leadership
  collaborative working model, 85*f*
  core partnership group, 86
  leading within and across partnerships, 84
  partner-leader skill components, 85*f*
  types, 84
Personal development plan (PDP), 73; *see also* Leadership
Personal health and social education (PHSE), 38
Personal skills, 29
PESTLE analysis, 54; *see also* Healthcare public health
Policy, 26
Population attributable fraction (PAF), 180
Population attributable risk (PAR), 180
Population healthcare, *see* Healthcare public health
Positive predictive value (PPV), 180
Post-test probability, 181
Precision, 181
Pre-test probability, 181
Prevalence, 181
Preventable fraction, 182
Prioritisation, 48
Programme budgeting, 50; *see also* Healthcare public health
Project management, 83; *see also* Change management
Public health (PH), 89
  assessments, 87
  career, 67
  tip, 46, 50, 52
  team, 26, 29, 33
Public Health England (PHE), 1
Public Health Online Resource for Careers, Skills, and Training (PHORCaST), 93
Public Health Skills and Knowledge Framework (PHSKF), 92; *see also* Public health assessments
  academic public health, 94
  care quality, 94
  collaborative working, 93
  health improvement, 93
  health intelligence, 94
  health protection, 93
  intervention efficacy assessment, 93
Purchasing power parity (PPP), 181
p value, 180

Q

Quality adjusted life year (QALY), 49, 182

R

Rate, 182
Rate ratio, 182
Re-orientating health services, 32
Relative risk (RR), 182
  reduction, 183
Reliability, 183
Repeatability, 183
Return on investment (ROI), 42
Risk, 7, 183
  ratio, 183

S

"Safe enough," 8
Scarcity, 48, 50
Scenario 1 (Human cadaver hazards), 101; *see also* Scenario feedback form; Video scenario
  candidate pack, 101–103
  examiner pack, 104–105
  role player briefing pack, 106–108
  scenario feedback form, 109, 159–160
Scenario 2 (Land contamination), 110–116, 161–162; *see also* Scenario feedback form; Video scenario
  candidate pack, 110–112
  examiner pack, 113–114
Scenario 3 (Human papilloma virus (HPV) vaccine), 117–123, 163–164; *see also* Scenario feedback form; Video scenario
  candidate pack, 117–119
  examiner pack, 120–121
  role player briefing pack, 122
  scenario feedback form, 123, 163–164
Scenario 4 (Interview on speed cameras), 124–131, 165–166; *see also* Scenario feedback form; Video scenario
  candidate pack, 124–126
  examiner pack, 127–128
  role player briefing pack, 129–130
  scenario feedback form, 131, 165–166
Scenario 5 (Exceptional funding request), 132–138, 167–168; *see also* Scenario feedback form; Video scenario
  candidate pack, 132–134
  examiner pack, 135–136
  role player briefing pack, 137
  scenario feedback form, 138, 167–168
Scenario 6 (Breast screening uptake rates), 139–145, 140t, 169–170; *see also* Scenario feedback form; Video scenario
  candidate pack, 139–141

examiner pack, 142–143
role player briefing pack, 144
scenario feedback form, 145, 169–170
Scenario 7 (Emergency hospital admissions), 146–151, 171–172; *see also* Scenario feedback form; Video scenario
candidate pack, 146–147
examiner pack, 148–149
role player briefing pack, 150
scenario feedback form, 151, 171–172
Scenario 8 (Smoking ban), 152–158, 153t, 173–174; *see also* Scenario feedback form; Video scenario
candidate pack, 152–153
examiner pack, 154–155
role player briefing pack, 156–157
scenario feedback form, 158, 173–174
Scenario feedback form; *see also* Video scenarios
Scientific and Technical Advisory Cell (STAC), 13
Screening, 14; *see also* Health protection
Secondary attack rate, 183
Sensitivity, 184
Severe acute respiratory syndrome (SARS), 8
Social marketing, 42
Social media, 18–19; *see also* Health protection
Soil guideline values (SGVs), 8
Source-pathway-receptor model, 11
Specificity, 184
Stages of change model, 30–32
Stakeholder; *see also* Healthcare public health
analysis, 53–54
communicating with, 60*t*–61*t*
desired shift for, 57*t*
map, 57*f*
and their involvement, 55*t*–56*t*
Statistically significant, 184
Statistical neighbours, 184
Steiner, Claude, 40
Strengths, weaknesses, opportunities and threats (SWOT), 54; *see also* Healthcare public health
of new vaccination programme, 58*f*
Stress management, 39–40; *see also* Health promotion
Structure of Healthcare Systems, 58
Supportive community, 29; *see also* Health promotion

T

Talking to the public, 16
Teenage pregnancy, 36*t*; *see also* Health promotion
Texas sharpshooter effect, 12; *see also* Health protection
360°feedback, *see* Multi-source feedback
Three-stage model of change, 74; *see also* Change management
Triage, 14; *see also* Health protection
Tuberculosis (TB), 2

U

UK Public Health Register (UKPHR), 92
UK public health specialty training, 91
competency key areas for, 92
curriculum, 91–92
Uncertainty and conflict, 37, 59

V

Vaccine efficacy, 184
Video scenarios, 95, 97; *see also* Scenario feedback form
breast screening uptake rates, 139
emergency hospital admissions, 146
exceptional funding request, 132
HPV vaccine to prevent cervical cancer, 117
interview on speed cameras, 124
infection hazards of human cadavers, 101
land contamination in a residential area, 110
marking criteria for Part B MFPH, 98*t*–100*t*
smoking ban, 152
utilization of, 97

Z

Zones at an incident, 14*f*

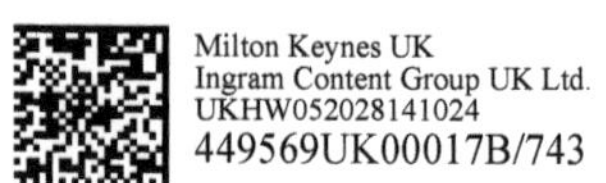

Milton Keynes UK
Ingram Content Group UK Ltd.
UKHW052028141024
449569UK00017B/743